I THINK I'M HAVING A
HEART ATTACK

I THINK I'M HAVING A
HEART ATTACK

By
Jerry Bishop

DOW JONES BOOKS
Princeton, New Jersey

This publication is designed to provide accurate and authoritative information in regard to the subject matter covered. It is sold with the understanding that the publisher is not engaged in rendering medical or other professional service. If medical advice or other expert assistance is required, the services of a competent professional person should be sought.

LCCN 74-17253
ISBN 0-87128-500-2
Copyright 1974

Preface

It seems incredible that heart attacks were not "officially" described before 1912 and then by a practicing physician in Chicago, Dr. J. B. Herrick. As a medical student in 1921, I was unaware of such a condition. People just didn't have "coronaries," or so one supposed. The infections, pneumonia, typhoid fever, syphilis and the like captured our attention. This lasted until Fleming and Florey discovered penicillin and with one giant blow changed the character of the practice of medicine, the insurance tables and the number of older people to care for!

The past decade has seen a remarkable change in the diseases physicians treat.

Now everyone agrees that heart attacks, hypertension and strokes are the major causes of disability and death. There is no longer a need to dwell on such a lugubrious fact, but for a few decades, relatively flamboyant methods were necessary just to get people's attention. Now that they are alive to it, what is to be done about it?

This is where Jerry Bishop comes in. Bishop is one of the soundest and most scholarly reporters of things medical and scientific in a field now grown large and sophisticated. I do not say such things lightly, if only because he has tough competition.

What you will read in "I Think I'm Having a Heart Attack" is how a highly informed layman sees heart attacks—probably as you will see them. Heart attacks have an unhappy way of occurring without notice and their results may be devastating. When physicians first began to study them seriously the outlook was gloom and doom. Now we know better. Many of us have had a heart attack—I am one—and live as long as we are statistically entitled to and enjoy most every minute of it.

There is a great tendency to think that a heart attack will never happen to *me*. For those who believe this, I recommend reading the obituary columns of any newspaper and a visit to any summer vacation spot. The first is tiresomely repetitive and the latter has become a modern day matriarchy of widows.

It is not enough to be prepared for an acute attack. Prevention should begin long before with a prudent lifestyle from childhood on. Our modern "abundant life" is a caution. From a generation of observing the abuse most people give their hearts, I can say if they don't have a coronary, they ought to!

And there is great need for people to learn to behave sensibly when a heart attack occurs. It often is the first occasion for the individual seriously to enter the medical world. It may be frightening unless you know the kind of thing Bishop tells you.

A heart attack is a family affair. So unannounced is the attack that there is no telling who will be available to help. Even more of a family affair does it become during the period of physical recovery and restoration of mental confidence.

If you join the company of the people who have had a heart attack and survived, where do you go from there? A long period of education and rehabilitation properly used can lead to a happy outcome. This book stresses such education because if you understand something of the nature of your ailment, it will help you enormously in knowing what to do and why.

Irvine H. Page, M.D.

Irvine H. Page, M.D. Scientist and statesman, Dr. Irvine H. Page is one of America's best-known and most-honored physicians. He is internationally recognized for his research in hypertension, arteriosclerosis and brain chemistry, and famed for his discovery of angiotensin and serotonin, which he and his associates later synthesized.

Contents

I.	The Coronary	1
II.	The Checkup	13
III.	Calculating the Odds	23
IV.	The Cholesterol Controversy	31
V.	Lowering the Pressure	41
VI.	Obesity: A Lost Cause?	53
VII.	The Psyche and the Heart	63
VIII.	When It Happens	71
IX.	Limiting the Damage, a New Theory	78
X.	Coronary Cinema	89
XI.	By-Passing the Coronaries	96
XII.	The Surgeon	104
XIII.	After the Attack	113
XIV.	A Patient's Chronicle	119
XV.	In the Future, a New Heart	129
XVI.	The Turning Point	137
	Glossary	141

I

The Coronary

At the very top of the heart, where the great artery or aorta that feeds blood to the entire body begins, there are the openings of two tiny blood vessels, their diameters no bigger than that of a pencil. One of these vessels emerges from the left side of the base of the main artery and makes its way down the outside of the heart, sending out tinier and tinier branches until the entire left side of the heart is covered with an intricate network of blood vessels. The other vessel similarly emerges from the right side of the aorta and enmeshes the right side of the heart. A microscope would reveal there isn't a part of the entire heart muscle that isn't reached by these two arterial nets.

To the anatomist and physiologist, Galen, who studied these two networks of arteries, or at least what he could see of them, they resembled a lacy crown for the heart, a *corona* in Latin. Hence, he called them the coronary arteries.

[Galen who practiced and taught in Rome in the Second Century A.D., also realized the ancient Greek anatomists had erred when they named the blood vessels arteries, which is the Greek word for "air holders." The Greeks had studied the body after death when the arteries are empty of blood and had assumed the vessels were air conduits. Galen

1

realized the arteries were filled with blood and that the heart had something to do with moving the blood. However, Galen's theories on where blood came from and where it went were so erroneous but so widely accepted that he effectively stifled cardiovascular research for 1,500 years.]

Galen, by all accounts, was somewhat of a showoff; he gave public demonstrations of his skills in anatomy and physiology using pigs and Barbary apes, the dissection of human bodies being illegal at the time. But even he couldn't have envisioned the extent to which his nomenclature for these two webs of arteries would be used. Today, 18 centuries later, there are few Americans who don't know someone who has suffered and perhaps died of "a coronary." The words "coronary occlusion" or "coronary thrombosis" or simply "coronary artery disease" probably appear on more hospital charts and death certificates than any other medical diagnosis.

The coronary arteries certainly deserve their rather regal name. The heart is a simple muscle and like any muscle requires a blood supply. Even though 4,300 gallons of blood flow through its four chambers every day, it cannot soak up its blood supply from its interior. It is the coronary arteries, tapping into the blood flow immediately after it leaves the heart, that nourish the heart muscle. Although the coronary arteries make up only a miniscule fraction of the 60,000 or so miles of blood vessels that weave through the body they are perhaps the most vital. If the coronaries fail to get blood, with its life-sustaining oxygen and nutrients, to any part of the heart muscle then that part of the muscle quickly dies, impairing, perhaps fatally, the ability of the heart to pump the same life-sustaining blood to the rest of the body.

The coronaries are the site of one of the most insidious and enigmatic diseases known to modern medicine. This is atherosclerosis, or simply, coronary artery disease, the clogging of the coronaries by fatty deposits on the walls of the arteries. It is insidious because it begins silently and progresses relentlessly for years, perhaps decades, before it makes its presence known in the form of a sudden and terrifying vice-like chest pain called a heart attack. It is enigmatic because medical scientists don't know how or why it begins or how to cure it.

Atherosclerosis isn't a new affliction. Evidence of it has been found in Egyptian mummies, including the mummy of a fat, old man, King Merneptah, who was pharaoh at the time of the Hebrew Exodus. And there are descriptions of fatal heart attacks as long ago as 2500 B.C.

But atherosclerosis in the past four or five decades has begun to appear in truly pandemic proportions, particularly in the United States and Western Europe; it is to the 20th Century American what tuberculosis was to the 19th Century American. Today an estimated 3,870,000 Americans currently have symptoms of the disease, the American Heart Association says. Unknown millions of others —perhaps every adult American—undoubtedly are afflicted with it in its symptomless stages. The result is that more than 675,000 die each year of a fatal heart attack, twice as many as die of cancer; indeed, heart attacks now account for more than a fourth of all deaths in the United States.

Heart researchers in the last 30 years or so have pieced together a detailed, albeit far from complete, picture of coronary artery disease and its end result, the heart attack.

It begins with the appearance of a fatty yellow streak appearing on the smooth inner lining of the coronary artery. Such fatty streaks can be found in the coronaries of most American males over age 20 and most females over age 40 (a clue that women may be protected by their sex hormones until menopause). Some kind of tissue reaction to this deposition sets in and the cells of the inner lining begin to proliferate creating a lesion or plaque. More and more fat from the blood, particularly a fatty substance called cholesterol, begins to accumulate in what is becoming a rough scar in the wall of the artery. The process of fat deposition and cell proliferation continues and the plaque grows larger, steadily narrowing the inside diameter of the artery at that spot.

The buildup may go on for 30 or 40 years without any noticeable symptoms. But as the deposit grows and the channel narrows, the amount of blood that can get past the deposit slowly decreases. The heart muscle lying downstream, which depends on the artery for an adequate blood supply, slowly becomes endangered.

Of all the organs in the body, the heart is the most sensitive to the amount of oxygen supplied by the blood. The kidney or the brain or the liver extract only about 10% to 25% of the total oxygen in the blood as it passes through. But the heart muscle needs 75% of the oxygen carried by the blood that flows through the coronary arteries. Thus, an adequate blood flow is of critical importance to the life of the heart muscle and its ability to do work.

For many people, the first symptom that some branch of a coronary artery has become dangerously narrowed may be a chest pain after heavy exertion or exercise. The exertion forces the heart to work harder and its oxygen needs go up sharply. The part of the heart muscle served by the partially clogged artery can no longer get enough blood to meet its increased needs, hence the chest pain as the heart muscle gasps for oxygen. The pain disappears upon rest when the oxygen demand drops back to a point that can be supplied by the amount of blood that is able to get through the narrowed artery.

This is a condition called angina pectoris, meaning a quinsy or kind of strangulation of the chest, a name picked for the syndrome in the 1700's before physicians realized it was related to what was then called "ossification" of the coronary arteries. Angina pain begins developing when a segment of a coronary is well over half closed, perhaps 75% or 80% narrowed, by atherosclerosis. As the clogging progresses, angina pain becomes more frequent; it can be triggered by climbing stairs or by excitement or anger. It can reach the point where even the exertion of getting out of bed can cause angina pain and some people become totally disabled by it.

In contrast to angina pectoris the heart attack is a sudden, unexpected event. But the same phenomena that underlie angina pectoris underlie the heart attack. The coronaries are narrowed by the atherosclerosis though, perhaps, the blood flow through the diseased artery is still adequate to meet the heart muscle demands even after heavy exertion. Suddenly, however, the diseased artery closes up or occludes completely, a "coronary occlusion," as it's called.

The heart muscle downstream is completely deprived of its blood—a situation called ischemia—and without oxygen this patch of muscle quickly loses its ability to pump blood by contracting. Unless the blood supply is restored in 30 minutes or an hour, the afflicted muscle cells die and the damage is permanent. The patch of heart muscle that dies is called an infarct and, since the heart muscle is known as the myocardium, the event is called a myocardial infarction.

If the sudden blockage occurs in one of the smaller branches of a coronary artery, only a relatively small amount of heart muscle may be injured. Indeed, a person may pass it off only as a severe case of heartburn. Blockage in a larger segment, however, results in a larger area of damage and a more painful attack, a pain often described as being like a squeezing of the chest.

Medical researchers aren't sure they know fully how a

coronary artery suddenly occludes. Sometimes, it seems, the diseased artery goes into a kind of spasm and the already narrowed channel clamps closed. In the majority of cases, however, it's believed the final plugging of the clogged artery is a blood clot, or a thrombus (hence, the term, coronary thrombosis).

Where the blood clot comes from is uncertain. Whether it formed on the spot or formed elsewhere and was washed into the diseased artery to lodge against the plaque isn't known.

Whether a person survives this sudden blockage of a coronary artery depends on how much of the heart muscle is damaged. If the occlusion blocks off the blood supply to more than, say, a quarter of the entire heart muscle, the heart simply can no longer work; it can't pump sufficient blood into its remaining open coronary arteries for its own survival much less get enough blood to the brain and the rest of the body. With such massive damage death is sudden and almost immediate.

With lesser damage this danger recedes although in severe heart attacks the threat of "pump failure" may exist for many hours after the initial pain strikes.

There are other problems that can beset the heart in the minutes and hours following the occlusion. One of the most common is the development of an irregular heart beat, an arrhythmia. The heart beat is controlled by electrical impulses, generated within the heart itself, that cause the heart muscle fibers to contract and, after the impulse wave passes, to relax. The impulses move in a wave through the heart muscle causing the muscle fibers to contract "in step" with their neighbors. Every fraction of a second a new wave of impulses starts moving through the heart muscle to produce the rhythmic 72 beats a minute of the heart.

When some of the muscle fibers are suddenly deprived of

6

oxygen by the heart attack, their ability to contract is severely affected. Some of the fibers may begin contracting completely out of step with other muscle fibers with the result that contractions of the heart become completely uncoordinated, a situation called fibrillation. Or the damaged heart may develop a rapid beat of more than 100 contractions a minute (tachycardia) or it may fall to an abnormally slow beat of less than 60 contractions a minute (bradycardia). These irregular heart beats if severe and prolonged can lead to death, particularly if they develop in the lower left chamber of the heart. It is this chamber, the left ventricle, that is responsible for pushing blood through the body's arteries and, thus, has to be the strongest and most efficient section of the heart.

Fortunately, 80% of the people who have their first heart attack survive (the odds go down sharply for subsequent heart attacks). The outward symptoms for a mild heart attack may be nothing more than feeling quite tired and distressed for a few days. For most heart attacks, however, the signal is a severe chest pain, right below the breast bone. The pain is variously described as crushing, constricting, or squeezing. The person will be pale, in a cold sweat and his breathing will be labored. If it weren't for the overriding impact of the chest pain, he probably would feel extremely tired. And, of course, he is frightened and anxious.

Strangely, it wasn't until 1912 that an American physician, Dr. James B. Herrick, actually gave a definitive description of the symptoms of a heart attack, and how it could be diagnosed. Until that time, most doctors had thought that a sudden obstruction of the coronaries was immediately and inevitably fatal and that if a person were alive he certainly wasn't suffering an obstruction of the coronaries.

It was another 10 to 20 years before medical researchers began developing an understanding of coronary artery disease and not until the late 1930's and the 1940's that scientists began developing ideas of what might be done about it. Even then their efforts were relatively meager, devoted largely to learning how to diagnose coronary artery disease and discovering its prevalence.

In the past two decades, however, research on coronary artery disease—indeed, on all cardiovascular diseases—has sharply expanded. Some public health officials place the turning point about the time of President Eisenhower's heart attack in September, 1955. The tremendous publicity on what had happened to the President—and the fact that he recovered—suddenly woke up the American public to the dangers and rising incidence of the disease. The result was that millions of dollars began pouring into the research laboratories.

The American Heart Association, in the 1954–55 fiscal year collected enough money to spend about $2.8 million on research; in the 1972–73 year it spent $16.8 million on cardiovascular disease research. The budget of the Federal government's National Heart & Lung Institute, at the same time, has increased several fold to nearly $300 million yearly.

There are hints that this expanding battle against coronary disease may be paying off. In early 1974, a new appraisal of the vital statistics on heart disease was published in the Journal of the American Medical Association by a Los Angeles heart specialist, Dr. Weldon J. Walker. By breaking down the death rates from "ischemic heart disease" into age brackets, Dr. Walker found that the death rate for middle-aged Americans may have peaked in 1963 and is now on the decline.

For instance, out of every 100,000 Americans aged 45–54, slightly more than 240 died of heart attacks or related ailments in 1963. This had dropped to 210 in 1969, the latest year for which accurate government statistics are available.

For the age group 55–64, the heart disease death rate dropped to 598 in 1969 from 668 only six years earlier.

It is only in people over 85 that the heart disease death rate has been rising for the past decade, Dr. Walker argues. In other words, although the overall death rate from coronary disease continues to rise, medicine may be effectively delaying an increasing number of fatal heart attacks to what might be called a more appropriate time of life. As one cardiologist puts it, "we're not trying to prevent death, only premature death."

It's most unlikely that Americans some morning will see banner headlines proclaiming the big breakthrough against coronary artery disease, at least not in the same way they read in 1955 that the Salk vaccine had been proven to be the breakthrough against polio. There is no evidence that coronary disease is caused by some virulent virus or bacterium and, thus, it isn't susceptible to the equivalent of vaccines and antibiotics that have conquered the infectious diseases.

Yet advances against coronary disease are occurring across a broad front, and though each one may not make front page news, they are starting to have a cumulative impact on the coronary pandemic.

By far the most important advances are the results of more than two decades of patient, painstaking studies of the differences between people who suffer and die of premature heart attacks and those who don't. These epidemiological studies are rapidly closing the circles of evidence convicting cigaret smoking, fat in the blood and diet, and high blood pressure as sharply boosting the risks of a premature heart attack. They also are focusing new scientific attention on the problem of obesity and the psychological aspects of heart attacks.

On the basis of these studies major public education campaigns are under way to convince Americans they ought to stop smoking, change their diet, and get their blood pressures down to normal. In noting the fact that heart attack deaths among the middle-aged began to decline in 1964, Dr. Walker said "The Surgeon General's Report on Smoking and Health and the vigorous educational program against risk factors by the American Heart Association coincided with the onset of the change in mortality trend."

Equally important, the epidemiological studies are turning that once-lackadaisical procedure, the annual checkup, into an increasingly powerful weapon against coronary disease. Given the silent nature of coronary disease the yearly examination of a seemingly healthy patient in the past gave precious little information about his risk of having a heart attack. Today, however, few physicians will fail, in such a checkup, to run a test for cholesterol in the blood, inquire into the patient's smoking habits, diet and lifestyle, and examine with a more knowing eye the electrocardiogram and chest X-rays. Even the routine measurement of blood pressure is taking on critical new importance with the growing knowledge of hypertension's role in heart attacks and stroke and the availability of drugs that can effectively lower high blood pressure.

Even if these preventive measures are totally successful, there will remain a large reservoir of coronary disease among Americans. Thus, the heart attack will continue to be a major problem for Americans and their doctors for years to come, though hopefully a diminishing problem.

It is in the treatment of the heart attack and the closely related angina pectoris that medical researchers are making some dramatic gains. There is, for example, the seemingly obvious but, until recently, almost insurmountable problem of getting a heart attack victim under medical treatment within the hour after the first chest pains strike. The number of heart attack deaths traceable to delays in getting to the hospital run in the tens of thousands. Now, however, a growing number of cities are operating emergency coronary ambulances with medically-trained crews that can reach a victim in minutes. The number of lives they've saved is starting to mount impressively.

Once in the hospital, the chances of a heart attack victim walking out again are showing spectacular increases. The widespread use of the new coronary care wards with their batteries of electronic monitors that can bring doctors and nurses rushing in at the first hint of arrythmias is cutting the in-hospital death rate from heart attacks in half. In the near future this death rate may even decline further with the recent discovery that the heart attack isn't a "bang-and-it's-over" phenomenon but, rather, that it may quietly continue for hours or even days. This discovery is triggering a whole new area of research that could lead to entirely new treatments of the heart attack.

For the first time, the surgeon's knife is being effectively wielded against coronary disease. Thanks to a new X-ray technique that can make the disease-clogged coronary arteries visible, more than 40,000 people a year are now undergoing surgery to bring in a new blood supply to hearts endangered by coronary disease. And at least one large research team in California is quietly perfecting that most dramatic of all operations, the transplant of a new heart.

This book is an attempt to describe these advances and where they stand at the moment. It isn't intended to report every recent development or detail in the long battle against coronary disease but, hopefully, it does pinpoint those advances which are having a significant impact against this most prevalent of all killing diseases.

Much of the material presented in the following pages is based on articles appearing initially in the Wall Street Journal which, for several years, has consistently chronicled the progress of medical science against coronary disease. Special acknowledgements should go not only to the Journal's editors but to several of its staff reporters whose articles are cited here. Richard D. James who spent a fascinating several days in 1969 with an open-heart surgeon wrote the original story that constitutes Chapter XII while the distressing discovery about obesity reported in Chapter VI is the work of David Brand. Part of the report on coronary by-pass surgery in Chapter XI is based on stories by Jonathan Spivak. Other reporters who contributed to this book include James F. Carberry, David P. Garino, and William M. Carley.

Odds are that the reader or some member of his or her family will encounter the frightening problem of coronary disease at some time or other. There should be no temptation, of course to rely on this book as a medical guide or as a basis for decisions that are better made by a physician. By necessity, a volume such as this, written by and for laymen, omits a vast amount of information and detail about coronary disease and certainly cannot substitute for the experience of a physician.

Nevertheless, the prevalence of coronary disease makes of it intense concern to everyone, whether it affects them directly or not. Perhaps an awareness of what the disease is and where scientists now stand in their effort to conquer it, will make it less frightening, less mysterious, and more manageable.

II

The Checkup

The room is small and quiet and the young lady is blonde and comely. As the man lies there, she places a cool hand on his forehead, looks into his eyes and says gently, "Look up and don't blink."

What follows is hardly a romantic interlude, for the young lady's interest in the gentleman is strictly clinical. She is a medical technician administering a tonometer test, the placing of a small cylindrical gauge on the dome of the eyeball to measure its resistance to pressure. Its purpose is to test for evidence of glaucoma.

The tonometer test is part of a comprehensive health examination or what most people might call a yearly checkup. In this instance it's administered about mid-way through a four-hour-long checkup given by technicians and physicians of a Manhattan organization that has been offering periodic health examinations to New Yorkers for more than half a century. Preceding and following the tonometer tests are X-rays, blood and urine analyses, electrocardiogram, lung tests and a host of other procedures all aimed at finding telltale signs of man's more common afflictions, ranging from cancer and heart disease to ulcers and gout.

The idea of a yearly health checkup is hardly new. Doctors have advocated it for decades—and most Americans have ignored it for as long. Only about a fourth of the population makes any attempt at all to get their health checked periodically and more than half the population has never had any such examination at all.

The periodic health examination, however, is being advocated with a growing urgency these days. One reason is strictly economic. A disease caught in its early, symptomless stages is considerably less costly to treat than in its advanced stages. With the costs of medical care skyrocketing and with an increasing proportion of these costs being borne by industrial and governmental health insurance plans, a rising number of employers, insurance companies, medical care plans and health authorities are trying to convince Americans to undergo periodic health checkups.

More important, though, the periodic health examination is designed to detect the incipient phases of the chronic diseases, the diseases that now account for the majority of deaths and disabilities. Heart disease, cancer and stroke account for 70% of all deaths in the nation. And health authorities estimate almost half of the population suffers from one or more chronic disorders ranging from arthritis and cataracts to diabetes and high blood pressure.

A periodic health examination does more than just spot a symptomless illness, however. Medical researchers in recent years have found various living habits and physical conditions which, while not diseases in themselves, do increase the risk of disease later. For example, high amounts of fats in the blood, smoking, and overweight are linked with an increased risk of heart attack. If nothing else, the annual checkup gives doctors a chance to spot such high-risk people and warn them away from their dangerous habits.

For most Americans who bother, the annual checkup is a

14

visit to the family doctor, followed by referral to a radiologist for X-rays and the submission of blood and urine samples to a medical laboratory.

For a small but growing number of people, however, the examination is performed at clinics specializing in health checkups. These may range from the posh and somewhat expensive Greenbriar Clinic in White Sulphur Springs, W. Va., a favorite of corporate executives, to the semi-automated examining clinics of the Kaiser-Permamente health plan on the West Coast where a subscriber can whisk through a score of examining stations in two or three hours with the results of each examination being immediately recorded and processed by computer.

For this reporter, the examination was done by the clinic in mid-Manhattan and it was, fortunately, a far cry from the ego-shattering "physical" that the Army inflicts on its inductees. In this case, it began, by appointment, at 10 a.m. with an attractive receptionist at the entrance to a large modernistic lounge not too different, perhaps, than the waiting room in a corporation's executive suite. Seated around the lounge were a number of men in thigh-length white cotton wrap-a-round smocks, regular suit trousers and street shoes. They aren't, as one first supposes, technicians and doctors waiting to pounce on the examinee but rather clients waiting their turn to visit the various examining rooms encircling the lounge.

After leaving my coat and shirt in a small dressing room and donning the white smock, I settle down in the lounge to the tedious task of filling out a medical history, a summary of past illnesses and accidents, family medical history, and notations on current living habits (smoking, drinking, diet, etc.) as well as physical complaints, if any. As annoying as the form-filling might seem, it is a key part of the examination. Later it will be studied and used as a guide by a physician in talking with the examinee about the results of the examination.

"Often, we can learn more from talking with a person than by examining him; if he's sick he's likely to tell us about it," explains one of the clinic physicians later. Thus, a note on the form about frequent headaches can be the clue for the physicians to query the examinee carefully about his manner of living, his working conditions and perhaps elicit from him other forgotten or unnoticed symptoms.

The first examination takes place in a stark, lead-lined room dominated by an awesome appearing X-ray machine. As per instructions, I hadn't had breakfast, not even a cup of coffee, in order for the stomach to be completely empty. Thus, the first "meal" of the day was a paper cup full of a pink, chalky liquid not unlike Pepto Bismol. The chalky liquid contains barium, a substance that being opaque to X-rays, will cast a shadow on the X-ray film. It will provide a detailed outline on the film of the stomach and duodenum or upper part of the small intestine, revealing any abnormal narrowings or obstructions.

Lying on the table underneath the X-ray machine, I try hard to heed the X-ray technician's instructions to "take a deep breath, hold it, don't move." Several X-rays are taken as I shift from one position to another.

Later, I'll return to the X-ray room for one last picture of the gastrointestinal tract. This is to see how much of the barium has moved from the stomach into the small intestine. "It normally takes about two hours for the stomach to empty," the doctor explains. "If we find the barium isn't emptying from the stomach at the normal rate, we'll wait a while and then take another X-ray." If it still appears the stomach is emptying unusually slowly, then suspicions are raised there is some obstruction in the duodenum, perhaps scar tissue from an ulcer or even a small tumor.

"We find ulcers in about 3% of the people we examine and in about a third of these there have been no symptoms," the physician says later. If an ulcer can be detected early enough it often can be treated with diet and antacids reducing the chances of it perforating the stomach or hemorrhaging.

A chest X-ray also is taken on the first visit to the X-ray room to look, of course, for spots on the lungs. "We don't see much tuberculosis anymore," the doctor says. But lung cancer is being seen increasingly frequently, notably among those whose medical history form indicates heavy cigaret smoking.

The chest X-ray also reveals in shadowy outline the size and configuration of the heart. The width of the normal heart is usually less than half the width of the chest. If it is larger it could be a sign the heart is being overworked because of atherosclerosis or other ills of the circulatory system.

"Enlarged hearts are frequently seen in conjunction with high blood pressure or overweight," the doctor explains. The enlarged heart shown on X-ray isn't always meaningful in itself. But when coupled with the blood pressure reading, the electrocardiogram, blood analyses and a medical history on smoking, eating and exercise habits, it can help uncover a person who might be at high risk of a heart attack.

After the X-ray room there is an embarrassingly long stop in the men's room to obtain a urine sample and use a self-administered disposable enema kit. Then there is a brief visit to another room to have a blood sample taken.

At the stop where the tonometer test for glaucoma is given, the attractive blonde also administers a sight test, a hearing test and an electrocardiogram. For the sight test, the classical chart on the wall long has been discarded. Instead, the examinee peers into an instrument, called an Orthorater, that resembles a binocular microscope. The machine displays a series of images that include not only the familiar lines of letters of decreasing size but also a series of geometric designs. The designs help uncover blind spots in the field of vision that could be the result of blood vessel hemorrhages caused by high blood pressure or diabetes.

The electrocardiogram is, perhaps, the most mysterious of the examinations. The examinee lies quietly on a padded table, wires attached to the ankles, wrists and chest, while the technician bends over a small machine on a nearby table, occasionally turning a knob with a loud click.

The procedure takes only a few minutes, is painless and requires nothing of the examinee except passivity. Yet, the electrocardiogram tends to be associated with providing the alarming confirmation of a damaged heart. Thus, as you lie on the table, staring at the ceiling you become acutely conscious of your heart beat and begin to wonder whether the wiggling pens are scratching out tell-tale signs of heart disease.

My curiosity about the results of the electrocardiogram was never fully satisfied. The electrocardiograph, that long sheet of squiggly lines, is one examination result the clinic physicians never show the client. The reason is that most laymen tend to overrate the capabilities of the electrocardiogram machine and too often they will misinterpret meaningless aberrations in the tracings.

The electrocardiogram only records the electrical impulses that ripple through the heart muscle causing it to contract. By attaching wires at different locations on the body, the machine can record the course of these impulses from different angles. If the impulses fail to follow their normal pathways or are arrhythmic this will show up as an abnormal tracing on the electrocardiograph.

Interference in the course of the impulses can be caused by a patch of muscle that has been or is being damaged because disease-clogged coronary arteries aren't providing a sufficient supply of blood. But a healthy heart also can produce a seemingly abnormal electrocardiograph—and a diseased heart may not produce any suspicious tracings at all. Thus, doctors caution, an abnormal electrocardiograph in an otherwise apparently healthy person is no more than a signal for more definitive tests and a doubly close look at the medical history (for mention of chest pains and other symptoms), the chest X-rays and other examination results.

Several minutes later, in another room, I find myself, trousers off, literally up-ended on a mechanically-elaborate tilting examining table for an examination by one of the proctologists, a pleasant, greying physician specializing in diseases of the rectum and colon. This proctological examination is one of the least talked about but most important of all, particularly in the over-40 age group. It's designed to detect polyps or growths in the lower intestine or large bowel.

Fortunately, the discomfort of the examination doesn't live up to pre-examination apprehensions. It is performed with the proctosigmoidoscope, a thin, hollow tube with a light at the end that can reach eight to ten inches into the bowel, past the rectum to the sigmoid colon or lower section of the colon.

The proctologist can peer down the tube and, with the aid of the lighted tip, look for polyps as he removes the tube. The area reached by the proctosigmoidoscope is the site of about 80% of the polyps ever found in the colon.

Polyps are found in 6% to 7% of the people examined at the clinic. Only a small fraction of these, however, are ever found to be malignant. Discovery of a cancerous polyp, though, is crucial. If found at an early enough stage they can be easily removed with a simple operation, thereby preventing a possibly fatal disease.

With the exception of a return to the X-ray room to check the clearance of the barium from the stomach, the examination ends with a visit to a physician for the physical checkup that is performed routinely in almost any physician's office. The examinee takes deep breaths while the doctor listens to the heart and lungs with a stethoscope; he coughs a few times as the doctor feels for signs of a hernia; lies on a table while he feels the abdomen for the size and tenderness of the spleen, liver and other organs (a large liver might be the sign of cirrhosis); blows on a whistle-like device to measure the capacity of the lungs (less than 4,000 cubic centimeters of exhaled air might be due to emphysema, asthma and/or smoking).

The mouth is inspected also but for more than just dental diseases. The physician also looks for leucoplakia, or tiny white spots on the lining of the mouth. These tiny spots, often found in smokers, can be pre-cancerous.

Behind the scenes, meanwhile, the blood and urine samples have joined those of hundreds of other examinees to be whisked to an automated clinical laboratory. These blood and urine tests are becoming increasingly comprehensive these days thanks to the advent of machines that can take a teaspoon of blood and run a dozen or more tests on it in a few minutes. "As long as you are going to do a few of the blood tests you might as well do them all since it costs only a few pennies more," says one preventive medicine specialist.

I'm asked to return a week later at 2 p.m. to see one of the clinic physicians to learn the results of the examination. There are occasionally moments in the intervening days when there are thoughts of shadowy X-rays revealing a glaring spot on the lungs or an electrocardiograph with a huge spike in the tracings that shouldn't be there. But after a half hour with the physician that afternoon, the fears are gone for everything appears to be normal.

The blood tests revealed a number of normal results. There were 15.7 grams of hemoglobin per 100 cubic centimeters of blood. A normal range, the physician explains, is 13 to 16 grams. The blood also consisted of 49% solids—a measurement called the hematocrit—and "anything above 40% is good." Had these measurements been abnormally low, they might have hinted at anemia.

The white blood cell count was 6,900 cells per cubic millimeter of blood, falling within the normal range of 6,000 to 10,000 cells. A high count here, the doctor says, would have hinted at an infection or, possibly, adult chronic leukemia, the kind of leukemia with which a person can live for many years if properly treated.

The amount of sugar in the blood, a check for diabetes, was 86 milligrams per 100 c.c. of blood whereas "anything under 120 milligrams is normal," he continues. There weren't any signs that the kidneys may be failing to remove urea nitrogen from the blood; the BUN, or blood urea nitrogen, measurement was 12 milligrams per 100 c.c. of blood, well below the 25 milligrams where doctors start to wonder if the kidneys are somehow damaged.

The amount of cholesterol in the blood was 189 milligrams per 100 c.c. "The average is about 230 milligrams and anything within 150 to 250 or so is acceptable," he explains. A high cholesterol level raises the risks of a heart attack. If the cholesterol level approaches 300 most doctors will advocate switching to a cholesterol-lowering diet, principally by changing the fat content.

The urine analysis showed no signs of either diabetes or kidney disease. The electrocardiograph was "within normal limits," and indicated the lower heart chambers to be in tune with the upper chambers, both beating at a rate of 77 beats per minute. The blood pressure pushed the little column of mercury on the sphygmomanometer up to 124 millimeters when the lower left chamber contracted (systolic pressure) and let it drop to 84 millimeters when the chamber relaxed (diastolic), for a reading of 124/84. What constitutes "normal" blood pressure varies widely among individuals although 100 to 140 systolic over 70 to 95 diastolic is thought to be normal.

It was only the medical history that brought any length of comment from the physician for it showed I smoked one to two packs of cigarets a day. This, for one thing, helped explain the notation of "congested mucous membranes" on the physical examination report. Noting that lung cancer is 10 times more common among smokers than non-smokers, the physician says I'm lucky to have gotten this far and still have a clear lung X-ray. "We haven't had a smoker with lung cancer yet who hasn't said he was sorry he didn't stop smoking years ago," the doctor says.

"If you find it impossible to stop smoking, at least try to cut down on it," he adds. "Put your cigarets in a different pocket each day. Then when you got to reach for them in the regular place and don't find them, it will be a reminder to tell yourself you can pass it up this time."

It is only later in looking at the written report that I noticed an item the physician apparently thought inconsequential. In the X-ray report describing an otherwise normal gastrointestinal tract it says "There is an inconstant spasm in the antral end of the stomach and bulb." I don't know what that is but so far I haven't found anyone else that has it.

III

Calculating the Odds

The ancient Romans, perhaps without realizing it, made a rather shrewd observation in the days when they were building their city on the wet and swampy plain surrounding the Tiber River: Those people who lived around the swamps were more likely to come down with intermittent fevers than those who lived elsewhere. The reason, obviously, was the bad air (*mal aria*) that swirled out of the swamps. The best way to reduce the risk of these fevers, they concluded, was to either move away to higher, drier areas, if one were rich enough, or to drain the swamps, which they did quite well.

Today, it's known that malaria is transmitted by mosquitoes which breed in the swamps. In addition to the use of insecticides, one of the most effective public health measures to combat malaria is to drain the swamps. In other words, the Romans, without knowing what was causing a disease, discovered an effective preventive measure.

This is the science of epidemiology in its most basic form. It is a science that already has proven a powerful tool in the eradication of many infectious diseases. It is now being wielded against coronary artery disease and the results are starting to push Americans into some major changes in their way of living.

23

I Think I'm Having a Heart Attack

It is a series of epidemiological studies that are uncovering links between coronary disease and smoking, high-fat diets, cholesterol, high blood pressure, family history and, even, perhaps, personality.

And it is another series of epidemiological studies, now underway, that will determine with finality whether changing the diet, stopping smoking and lowering blood pressure will reduce a person's risk of dying of a heart attack. If these studies turn out as most heart specialists predict, then Americans may well have the means of stemming the rising toll of coronary disease long before laboratory scientists can pin down exactly how it's caused. Indeed, many researchers believe this evidence is already at hand and that these newest studies are needed only to resolve, once and for all, the controversies that continue to flare around the epidemiology of heart disease.

Epidemiology is literally the study of the incidence and spread of a disease in a group of people, that is, the study of an epidemic. It, hopefully, turns up clues on how to stop the epidemic and to prevent it breaking out again in the future. Its methods involve comparing groups of people afflicted by a disease with similar groups of healthy people, searching for factors among the sick that are rare or non-existent among the healthy.

Epidemiologists quickly concede their science has a number of pitfalls and shortcomings. It cannot prove what causes a disease; it merely shows a statistical association between some factor and the disease. An epidemiologist rushing into a boarding school to investigate an outbreak of, say, hepatitis may find that all the sick students are also football players. This doesn't mean playing football causes hepatitis but only that there is some association. It is a clue to look further, perhaps checking the food served at the training table, or the drinking water in the locker room.

What's more, epidemiologists must go to elaborate lengths to make sure their results are "statistically significant." This means that statistical differences turned up by such studies must not result from chance coincidence alone. It is unlikely, for example, that one could examine 10 heart patients and 10 healthy persons and come up with any statistically significant differences; they might find six heart patients smoked and only four healthy persons smoked but this could be strictly a coincidence that could occur in any randomly picked group of 20 persons. Such a difference would have to occur in hundreds or perhaps thousands of people before it became statistically significant.

Most important, doctors caution, is that group differences uncovered by epidemiologists don't always apply to individuals. Not everyone who lives near a swamp gets malaria while some people who don't live near swamps do get it. It's just that swamp dwellers have a higher risk and they can lower their risks by moving away.

Bringing epidemiology to bear against coronary heart disease is difficult because, unlike a virus epidemic, heart disease develops over years or even decades. Hence, entire life histories of large groups have to be studied to spot statistically significant differences between heart patients and those without heart disease. And given the fact no two people are exactly alike nor do they live exactly the same way this is no easy task. For instance, differences in coffee consumption, television set ownership and drinking water hardness have been statistically linked with heart disease but the evidence is far from conclusive.

Nevertheless, such studies are starting to pay off and doctors are reaching the point where they can calculate the odds of a person having a heart attack with almost the accuracy a good poker player can calculate the odds of drawing a third ace.

I Think I'm Having a Heart Attack

One of the most successful of these studies is known informally as the Framingham study (formally as the Heart Disease Epidemiology Study). Around 1950, the National Heart Institute, a part of the U.S. Public Health Service, sent a team of physicians and epidemiologists into Framingham, Mass., a town about 20 miles from Boston picked as a fairly typical American community. In the ensuing four years they gave meticulous medical examinations and took careful medical histories of more than 5,000 adult volunteers in the town.

The researchers then closely watched what happened to these 5,000 adults. They provided medical checkups at least once every two years, checked hospital admissions, interviewed spouses and family physicians and studied death certificates. By the mid-1960's the statistics began developing significance. By 1968, for instance, almost 500 of the 5,000 adults had developed signs of coronary artery disease, usually either a heart attack or angina pectoris.

By looking at the medical records, the researchers began to spot differences between those who developed coronary disease and those who didn't. The risk of a heart attack among young men with high amounts of cholesterol in the blood when the study began was four to seven times higher than among a group of men of the same age who had low cholesterol levels.

Smokers who puffed more than one pack of cigarets daily had a three-fold greater incidence of coronary disease than non-smokers of the same age. Greater risks also were linked with high blood pressure, overweight and electrocardiogram abnormalities.

More important, any combination of these factors appeared to compound the risk of a heart attack. A smoker with high blood pressure and high cholesterol level ran a 12-fold greater risk of a heart attack than a non-smoker with normal blood pressure and low cholesterol levels.

More recently, an effort called the Pooling Project, undertaken by the American Heart Association, combined all the statistical data from not only the Framingham study but from similar studies of industrial workers in Chicago, businessmen in Minneapolis, civil servants in Los Angeles and Albany, N.Y., and a host of other groups. The project then measured the rates of first heart attacks during a 10-year period among white American males who were under 60 years old when the studies began. The figures leave little doubt what factors contribute to the risks of having a premature heart attack.

A high cholesterol level is one factor. Of each 1,000 men with cholesterol levels of 175 to 199, which is fairly low, there were 52 first heart attacks. The rate was double that among men with cholesterol levels between 250 and 300 and was tripled if the cholesterol level was over 300.

High blood pressure produced almost identical figures, with men having very high blood pressure having three times the rate of premature heart attacks as those with the lowest pressure.

Smokers of more than one pack of cigarets daily had three times the rate of premature heart attacks as non-smokers and twice that of men who smoked less than half a pack daily.

Any combination of these three risk factors boosts the chances of a premature heart attack dramatically. Among each 1,000 men who suffered all three risk factors there were 171 first heart attacks, or nine times as many as among men free of all three risk factors. Possessing only two of the risk factors, made it almost five times as likely to have a first heart attack as possessing none.

"These impressive findings indicate that these three risk

factors . . . are properly designated major risk factors for premature atherosclerotic heart disease, especially coronary heart disease," declares the Inter-Society Commission for Heart Disease Resources, a group of experts set up with Federal funds to lay out a national blueprint to combat heart disease.

Epidemiologists have uncovered several other possible risk factors in coronary disease but the evidence isn't yet as convincing as it is for smoking, cholesterol levels and high blood pressure. Diabetes appears to increase the risk but then many diabetics also suffer high blood pressure.

Coronary disease and heart attacks also are more common among overweight people but this may be because obese people tend to have high cholesterol levels, high blood pressure and diabetes. "Moderate overweight—in the absence of these risk factors and cigaret smoking—apparently is associated with only a modest increase in risk," the Inter-Society Commission notes.

To the high-caliber Inter-Society Commission the statistical evidence is strong enough to warrant launching a major national program to lower cholesterol levels by changes in the national diet, to eliminate cigaret smoking, and to get high blood pressure under control with drugs. The evidence, that these risk factors are the causes of heart disease, the commission concedes, isn't conclusive. But, it argues, "at times urgent public health decisions must be made on the soundest evaluation and best judgment of available incomplete evidence."

If such a national program could get every white male between 35 and 64 years old to stop smoking, lower his cholesterol and keep his blood pressure normal, then it would prevent 300,000 cases of coronary disease and 60,000 deaths annually, the commission calculates. Such effectiveness, of course, would be impossible to achieve. But, the group says, even if the program were only 50% effective among 50% of these men, it would still prevent 75,000 new cases of coronary disease and 15,000 deaths a year.

The impact, theoretically, would be greater than these figures indicate since many women and non-whites also would be affected by such a program. Unfortunately, almost all the epidemiological studies have been done among groups of white males since 20 years ago this was the group where the pandemic of premature heart attacks was breaking out.

But many medical experts argue that despite such promising estimates, the epidemiological studies still leave a major question unanswered.

"One thing is clear: statistical association must not be immediately equated with cause and effect," the editors of Lancet, the prestigious medical journal published in Britain, have warned. "To give proof of cause and effect between one risk factor and disease requires its isolation as a cause, and proof of benefit through its elimination," they noted.

"So far, despite all the effort and money that has been spent, the evidence that eliminating risk factors will eliminate heart-disease adds up to little more than zero in terms of preventing heart-disease on a public health scale," Lancet declared.

In other words, such medical analysts say, the real clincher will be to show that reducing or eliminating the risk factors actually does reduce the incidence of coronary disease and heart attacks.

It is to this end that the MR. FIT experiment has been launched. The initials stand for the Multiple Risk Factor Intervention Trial, a six-year-long, $10 million experiment funded by the National Heart and Lung Institute. In the initial phase of this experiment, medical teams will screen a half million American middle-aged men looking for 12,000 who are seemingly healthy but have a high risk of heart disease as determined by their cholesterol levels, smoking habits, and blood pressure.

All of these men will be told of their high risk profiles. But half will be referred to their own doctors for advice and help, that is, they'll be given the same help most Americans are currently given in regards to reducing the risks of heart disease. The other 6,000 men, however, will be enrolled in intensive programs to get their cholesterol levels down by diet or drugs, to bring their blood pressure back to normal and to get them to give up smoking. Hopefully, the medics can get at least a 40% reduction in smoking, and at least a 10% lowering of blood pressure and cholesterol levels—and keep it that way for the six years.

If, at the end of the experiment, the intensively-treated group has had significantly fewer heart attacks or other signs of heart disease than the conventionally-treated group, then epidemiologists believe they'll have both proof of cause-and-effect and the evidence to convince Americans to start changing their way of living.

IV

The Cholesterol Controversy

In the late 1950's advertisements began appearing in newspapers and magazines extolling the amount of polyunsaturated fats contained in various margarines, shortenings and other vegetable-oil-based foods. The inference was fairly clear: polyunsaturated fats help reduce the amount of cholesterol in the blood and in turn reducing cholesterol levels reduces the risk of a heart attack.

In late 1959, however, the ads were abruptly halted. The U.S. Food & Drug Administration warned the food processors that "any claim, direct or implied, in the labelling of fats and oils or other fatty substances offered to the general public that they will prevent, mitigate or cure diseases of the heart or arteries is false and misleading." In other words, the FDA said there was no evidence that cholesterol levels were related to coronary artery disease.

In late 1973, fourteen years later, a series of ads began appearing in the Wall Street Journal and the New York Times extolling the benefits of eating eggs. Paid for by the industry-financed National Commission on Egg Nutrition, the ads declared "There is absolutely no scientific evidence that eating eggs, even in quantity, will increase the risk of a heart attack."

31

I Think I'm Having a Heart Attack

This time it was the American Heart Association's turn to fume. Egg yolks are rich in cholesterol and cholesterol in the blood is definitely linked to heart disease, the association argued. In a petition to the Federal Trade Commission asking that the ads be halted, the association called them false and misleading.

Thus, the controversy over fats in the diet, cholesterol in the blood and coronary artery disease continues. But, as the incident with the egg ads indicate, it is a subtly different argument today than it was 15 or 20 years ago. Less and less is the claim challenged that there is a link between high cholesterol levels in the blood and a high risk of a heart attack. And there is little dispute that a high cholesterol level can be lowered somewhat by manipulating the diet, particularly by substituting polyunsaturated fats for animal fats.

Indeed, in the winter of 1973–74, at least one brand of margarine was being promoted solely on its content of polyunsaturated fats. The TV commercials openly claim that a diet high in polyunsaturates can lower cholesterol levels by 15%. The commercials failed to bring a murmur of protest from either the FDA or the FTC.

Instead the debate now centers on the final and most important question of all: Does lowering cholesterol levels by diet or with drugs actually reduce the risks of a heart attack—or is a person who is prone to high cholesterol levels inherently at a high risk of heart attack no matter what he does to lower his cholesterol level?

Cholesterol is a yellowish fatty substance that apparently is involved in the complex business of transporting and distributing fats throughout the body, and it may be one of the raw materials for hormones, including the sex hormones. It is manufactured naturally in the liver where it is hooked to a protein. This cholesterol-protein combination

32

is a vital component of all animal cells and is one of several kinds of fat-protein combinations that are found in the blood stream.

Although most of the cholesterol in the blood is made by the body, some does originate in the diet since cholesterol is an ingredient of all animal tissues, including steaks and eggs.

The evidence linking the diet, cholesterol and heart disease is largely circumstantial. It's been known for at least a century that cholesterol is a major ingredient of the deposits that clog the arteries in coronary artery disease. It's also been known since the 1900's that in animals, at least, a diet rich in cholesterol and fat, particularly animal fat, can lead to high cholesterol levels in the blood.

At the same time, epidemiologists many years ago noted that deaths from heart attacks among middle-aged men were far more common in countries consuming a high amount of animal fat than among people eating a low-fat diet. Many heart researchers think it is no coincidence that coronary artery disease has increased among Americans as their consumption of fats has gone up. The average American in 1910 got only about 32% of his calories from fats; today he gets 40% to 45% of his calories from fats—and he eats a lot more calories.

Studies such as the 20-year-long study in Framingham, Mass., have helped nail down the risk of high cholesterol levels. In that study, U.S. Public Health Service researchers measured the cholesterol levels of hundreds of men between the ages of 30 and 62 back in the early 1950's. They then watched for 15 years to see how many men developed heart attacks or other signs of coronary artery disease.

The results: Among men with cholesterol levels of 250 milligrams per 100 milliliters of blood or higher, the rate of heart attacks was almost three times the rate among men with levels of 194 milligrams or lower. Moreover, the risk rose proportionately to the cholesterol levels. Among men with readings between 221 and 249, the rate was twice that of the low-cholesterol men.

A person can load up his blood with cholesterol by eating foods containing cholesterol, itself. But many heart researchers believe strongly the most important culprit is the kind of fat as well as the amount of fat eaten. All fats contain so-called fatty acids of which there are two major kinds, saturated and unsaturated. This refers basically to whether the fatty acid molecule contains all the hydrogen atoms it can hold. If it does, it is saturated; if it is lacking one hydrogen atom it is monounsaturated and if it lacks two or more hydrogen atoms it is polyunsaturated.

Generally, saturated fatty acids are solid at room temperature while unsaturated fatty acids are liquid. Most animal fats—lard and butter, for instance—are composed of saturated fatty acids and hence are solid or "hard." Vegetable fats, such as cottonseed or soybean oil, are relatively high in unsaturated fatty acids and are liquid. (Unsaturated fatty acids tend to grab oxygen molecules from the air and go rancid; years ago food chemists learned they could increase the shelf life of vegetable oils by artificially hydrogenating them to produce a solid, saturated fat commonly called shortening).

It is a high amount of saturated or "hard" fat in the American diet that researchers believe is behind the high amount of cholesterol in the blood of the middle-aged American. About 42% of the fatty acids Americans consume is of the saturated type most of which comes from dairy products like milk, cheese and butter and from the fats in meat like the fat-marbled prime steaks and roasts Americans cherish. Of the rest of the fatty acids, about 41% are monounsaturated and only 17% are polyunsaturated, the latter coming mostly from vegetable oils and fish.

Notes the Inter-Society Commission for Heart Disease Resources "with very few exceptions human populations consuming diets high in saturated fat and cholesterol have high mean serum cholesterol levels and high incidence and mortality from premature CHD (coronary heart disease). Human populations consuming diets low in cholesterol and saturated fat have low mean serum cholesterol levels and low incidence and mortality rates from premature CHD."

For example, more than a dozen studies of heart disease deaths among middle-aged men in various countries showed the Finns and Americans at the top of the list and the Japanese at the bottom. The Finns and Americans eat a lot of animal fat, the Japanese don't.

Many researchers as well as the American Heart Association and the Inter-Society Commission believe the link between cholesterol in the blood and coronary heart disease is now strong enough to warrant major efforts to get Americans to bring their cholesterol levels down. The method, they argue, is to change the national diet, cutting back sharply on the saturated fat and cholesterol-bearing foods and substituting wherever possible the polyunsaturated fats.

It's been known for more than a decade that such manipulation of the diet can lower cholesterol levels. In the early 1960's at the Cleveland Clinic, for example, 25 married medical students and their spouses agreed to try out some special fat-modified foods for 10 months to see if their cholesterol levels were affected.

In this study, a local packer took special pains to trim off all visible fat from meats. A pork roast, which normally is about 20% fat was trimmed to 8% fat, for example. Frankfurters, baloney, liver sausage, breakfast sausage and ham loaf were all made from lean meats and cottonseed oil. Cheeses and ice creams were developed in which cottonseed and corn oils were substituted for butterfat. Similar substitutions for animal fats were made in chow mein, chili and pizza. Eggs were limited to five a week and pastries were made without egg yolks or saturated shortening.

The results: The average concentration of cholesterol in the blood of the husbands dropped more than 13% and in the wives about 15%.

It was such studies as this one that spurred heart researchers at that time to propose a grandiose experiment. They wanted to answer two major questions haunting the diet-cholesterol idea. One was whether it was practical to believe the American diet could be changed on a national scale. And, if Americans could change their diets, would it make any difference in the incidence of coronary heart disease?

The first question is of prime importance. If Americans are so wedded to their present high-fat diets they couldn't stick to the new cholesterol-lowering diets, there is little use of talking about changing the national diet. The answer comes from the National Diet-Heart Feasibility Study.

In the Diet-Heart Feasibility Study, 2,400 middle-aged American men in five cities and a mental institution were asked to go on special diets using foods prepared especially for the study by commercial food processors. The foods were supplied through special commissaries set up for the study. The foods, however, weren't identical. One group of men was supplied foods that closely approximated the average American diet, that is, about 40% of the calories were from fat, mainly saturated fat. Less than 7% of the total calories were from polyunsaturated fats. The amount of cholesterol eaten each day was about 650 to 750 milligrams.

Another group of men were given foods that yielded a cholesterol-lowering diet. The amount of cholesterol eaten each day was cut almost in half, to between 350 and 450 milligrams. Total fat eaten was reduced to 30% of calories and of this, the saturated fat intake was cut in half and the polyunsaturated fat intake was doubled.

The men on the cholesterol-lowering diet did, indeed, show an average drop in cholesterol levels of 11% to 12%. Not all the men were able to stick to the diet closely for two years but the 100 men who followed it most faithfully had cholesterol declines averaging 13.6%.

Even the men on the typical American diet showed some decline in cholesterol levels which, the researchers said, was because they had become conscious of the amount of fat they were eating and cut back voluntarily.

On the basis of this study, the Inter-Society Commission believes the American diet can be changed and cites some specific methods. In addition to getting rid of excess weight, the commission wants Americans to cut their cholesterol consumption in half, bringing it down to about 300 milligrams daily. This means such measures as limiting the consumption of egg yolks, the richest source of cholesterol, to about three or four a week. Eating of shellfish, another source of cholesterol, also would be reduced.

Overall fat consumption should be cut down to less than 35% of total calories, with only 10% of the calories coming from saturated fat, 10% from monounsaturated fat and 10% from polyunsaturated fat (up from less than 7%). This means eating lean steaks, roasts and other meats and using the "soft" margarines or the vegetable oils instead of butter, hydrogenated shortening and the like.

The commission wants meat packers to produce sausages, hot dogs, cold cuts and other processed meats in which the saturated animal fat has been partly replaced by polyunsaturated vegetable oils. The dairy industry is urged to develop low-cholesterol, low-butterfat milk and cheeses. (Ironically, changes in the fat content of processed meats and in milk will require changes in old laws that were passed to prevent adulteration of meats and watering of milk.)

The commission also urges Americans to eat more poultry and fish, and to go easy on organ meats such as liver. In short, no more bacon and eggs for breakfast or prime steak and chocolate eclairs for dinner.

If Americans were to change to this cholesterol-lowering diet, would it do any good? The Inter-Society Commission thinks so, of course. Its statisticians calculate that "a 5% reduction in serum cholesterol level of the U.S. population would yield a 12.8% decrease in CHD incidence while a 10% reduction in serum cholesterol level would result in a 24.4% decrease in CHD incidence."

But even the commission concedes there are "differences of opinion" over whether enough is known to warrant changing the national diet. So far, there have been only a few experiments that hint that lowering cholesterol levels cuts the risk of a heart attack. Two studies, one in Finland and one in a Veterans Administration hospital in Los Angeles, did show some reduction in the incidence of heart disease among people whose cholesterol levels were reduced by dietary means. But, as the epidemiologists say, the differences weren't "statistically significant."

Some other experiments using cholesterol-lowering drugs instead of diet, also hint at a reduction of risk of a heart attack. There are two or three such drugs available and doctors frequently prescribe them for people with relatively high cholesterol levels, particularly if they also have other "risk factors" such as overweight, a family history of heart disease, heavy smoking, etc.

The Cholesterol Controversy

One of these studies, using a drug called clofibrate or Atromid-S, involved 3,200 men and was conducted by physicians with United Air Lines in San Francisco. They found that in one group of more than 1,000 men, whose average age was 47.5 years, the non-fatal heart attack rate was 1.89 per 1,000 persons each year for men treated with the drug, but a significantly larger 6.6 per 1,000 each year for men who didn't get the drug.

In the same study, another group of 2,000 men, whose average age was 10 years younger, the apparent protection afforded by clofibrate against nonfatal heart attacks was even more dramatic: 0.64 per 1,000 among the treated men, five per 1,000 among the untreated men.

Strangely, the study didn't find any difference in the death rate for the treated and untreated men, only that the incidence of nonfatal heart attacks was markedly lower. The researchers at the time, early 1972, ascribed this to the fact that the study hadn't gone on long enough to get significant statistics on death rates. Even more puzzling is the fact that clofibrate wasn't effective in lowering cholesterol levels in several of the men but even their heart attack rate appeared to be lower.

The researchers who carried out the Diet-Heart Feasibility Study had wanted to launch what they believed would have been the definitive experiment to find out whether lowering cholesterol levels would reduce heart deaths. They proposed enrolling 68,000 men in the experiment. They would be divided into groups as closely alike in terms of age, cholesterol levels, weight, etc., as possible. Some groups would go on cholesterol-lowering diets, others wouldn't.

With 68,000 men involved, the statisticians estimated that within five years they would have statistically significant results as to whether the death rate was lower among men whose cholesterol levels were reduced by diet. With fewer men, it would take much longer to get significant results:

But in 1971 this idea was shelved in the midst of cutbacks in the Federal budget for heart disease research. The study would have cost anywhere from $80 million to $380 million, depending on just how large and elaborate it was.

In its place the National Heart and Lung Institute has launched the so-called MR. FIT study (for multiple risk factor intervention study). This will test not only the cholesterol theory but also see if reducing smoking and high blood pressure can reduce the risk of heart attacks. Men with all three risk factors will be enrolled. Attempts to bring down high cholesterol levels by diet and/or drugs will be coupled with attempts to eliminate smoking and lower blood pressures. The results of this experiment aren't expected to be known until at least 1977 and probably later.

"The public health importance of CHD makes it mandatory to conduct such trials," says the Inter-Society Commission. But, it adds, "even if planning were to start immediately (1972), the American public would probably have to wait at least 10 years for results of these studies." To wait this long before making a decision on the national diet is wasting time on a question of considerable public health urgency, the commission argues. The existing evidence, although incomplete, is still strong enough to justify changing the American diet to effect a lowering of cholesterol levels, it declares.

V

Lowering the Pressure

Medical scientists are starting to crack the mysteries of one of the most insidious and prevalent diseases in the nation: high blood pressure.

In laboratories around the country researchers are piecing together a picture of what goes awry in the body when the pressure of the blood rises to dangerously high levels and stays there. In the clinics, doctors are working out new, highly effective treatments for lowering blood pressure. And in the streets public health officials are mounting a major nation-wide campaign to discover and get under treatment literally millions of Americans who are unaware that their blood pressure is high enough to threaten their life.

High blood pressure, or hypertension, is exactly what it says, a condition in which the blood is being pumped through the vast network of arteries with unusually high force. It's difficult to say at what point the blood pressure rises from "normal" to "high," as measured by the column of mercury on the doctor's sphygmomanometer or blood pressure recorder. But generally physicians classify a person as hypertensive if his diastolic pressure—the smaller of the two-number pressure readings—is 95 millimeters of mercury or higher.

I Think I'm Having a Heart Attack

Everyone experiences temporary increases in blood pressure. Emotions can push up pressure for short periods, for instance. Indeed, a patient's apprehension about a blood pressure reading can raise his pressure a bit, which is why doctors usually insist on taking three readings in a two-week period before making a firm diagnosis of hypertension.

As late as the 1920's physicians didn't think high blood pressure was a threat to health. In fact, it was deemed a natural and necessary attempt by the body to keep sufficient blood flowing through arteries that were beginning to harden and narrow from age or disease.

In the last few years, however, researchers have developed hard evidence that high blood pressure, if left unchecked for a few years, sharply increases the risk of a heart attack, heart failure or a stroke leading to disability and/or death. Epidemiological studies such as the Framingham study, for instance, show the rate of heart attacks among men whose diastolic pressure was 105 or higher was more than twice that of men with pressures of less than 95 and three and a half times that of men with pressures of less than 85 millimeters of mercury.

More important, researchers only recently have added the final bit of evidence proving that hypertension is a threat to life. They showed that by lowering high blood pressure the risk of death or disability also dropped.

In what is now hailed as a turning point in hypertension research, a group of Veterans Administration hospitals selected more than 500 men who had high blood pressure. Half of the men were assigned to receive drugs that lowered their pressure, the other were given placebos or inert pills.

The VA doctors, under the chairmanship of Dr. Edward D. Freis, then watched carefully to see, first, if the drugs could effectively hold down blood pressure for periods of years, and, second, if they do any good in preventing death. The study was supposed to last five years. But in the men with extremely high pressures—115 and higher—the differences were strikingly evident in the first two years. Among this group of 143 men, the half receiving placebos suffered four deaths, at least three of which were due to bursting of the aorta or major artery. Moreover, 17 other men in this untreated group developed such serious complications of hypertension they had to be pulled out of the study and put under treatment.

By contrast, in the treated half of this extremely high-pressure group there weren't any deaths and only two men who developed complications; one man had a stroke and another suffered adverse reactions to the drugs. As a result, the VA doctors ended the experiment for all of these extremely high pressure men after the first two years.

For the remaining 380 men with less severe hypertension, however, the study continued the full five years and by 1970, the doctors had the answer. Among the untreated men, 19 died, most of the deaths being due to stroke or congestive heart failure. Another 16 developed medical problems due to the high blood pressure, at the first sign of which, the doctors withdrew them from the study and put them under active treatment.

Among the men whose blood pressures had been brought down by drugs, there were only eight deaths and only one man had to pull out of the study because, following a heart attack, he couldn't tolerate the drugs.

To medical researchers the VA study clinched the case that lowering high blood pressure would dramatically reduce the risk of a stroke or congestive heart failure. The differences in heart attacks between untreated men and the men whose pressure was brought down wasn't statistically significant, however. The reason, it's thought, is that the 500 men picked for the study had fairly severe hypertension and had had it for quite a long time. Thus they were most likely to succumb to the direct effects of high blood pressure such as bursting arteries that produce strokes before the hypertension could exert its effect on the heart.

The VA is now launching a similar study among 8,000 patients who are a bit younger and who have milder hypertension. The aim is to see if lowering the pressure in the early stages will slow down the clogging of the coronary arteries by atherosclerosis, and thus reduce the risk of a heart attack.

Contrary to popular belief, hypertension isn't a disease of old age. A study by New York's Presbyterian Hospital Hypertension-Nephritis Clinic a few years ago of several hundred hypertensives found that the disorder was first detected at a mean age of 32, which means that half of the patients developed high blood pressure before this age. Among these untreated hypertensives, death occurred on the average about 20 years after their high blood pressure was discovered, although some patients lived for as long as 40 years afterwards.

About 7% of these patients developed what is called malignant or, perhaps more accurately, accelerated hypertension. This is where a patient might go along for years with his elevated pressure staying fairly constant. Then, suddenly for no apparent reason, it starts going up higher and higher. If untreated, this form is often fatal in a year or two.

The vast majority of Americans with high blood pressure are classed as suffering "essential hypertension." This means the cause of hypertension isn't known, that no matter how closely the patient is examined doctors can't find any abnormality that would cause a sustained high blood pressure. In only a few hypertensives, perhaps only a tenth, are physicians able to spot a tumor, an injury or a disease that would cause the body to maintain an abnormally high pressure.

The unknown cause of most hypertension is a major obstacle to finding a cure. Fortunately, chemists in the last several years have developed a variety of drugs that can lower blood pressure to normal or near-normal levels. But these drugs aren't curing the basic defect and, thus, they have to be taken for life.

Hypertension researchers, however, believe they may now be on the track to uncovering the cause—or causes—of high blood pressure. The body has several ways of raising and maintaining blood pressure; if it didn't a person who suddenly stood up after lying down for a while would faint since there wouldn't be enough pressure to get blood to the brain against the pull of gravity. Presumably, in hypertension, something has gone wrong with these pressure-maintaining mechanisms.

It's known that one of these pressure-maintaining mechanisms lies with the nervous system. Tiny nerves around the blood vessels can tighten up, constricting or narrowing the blood vessels. The effect is like tightening the nozzle on a garden hose. To get the same amount of water—or blood—through the much narrower opening, the pressure must increase.

The nervous system, is thought to be the mechanism that makes the quick response to the body's sudden need for a change in blood pressure. It reacts when monitoring points called barostats, scattered throughout the blood system, detect a drop in blood pressure. There are barostats in the two main arteries in the neck that supply blood to the brain, for example. When they detect a drop in pressure that threatens the brain, they signal the nervous system to raise pressure, it's believed.

45

One theory is that a person who reacts strongly to emotional stresses may be repeatedly triggering the nervous system to raise his pressure. Eventually, it's theorized, the barostats, being hit time after time with this higher pressure begin to consider it normal and, consequently, are "reset" to maintain the higher level of pressure.

More recently, scientists' attention has been turning to another pressure-maintaining mechanism. This is a chemical mechanism and, from an evolutionary viewpoint, is apparently more primitive than the nervous system mechanism. Its central control lies in the kidney.

Researchers discovered years ago in experiments with dogs that when the main artery supplying blood to the kidney is clamped shut, causing a drop in blood pressure in the kidney, the pressure throughout the rest of the body starts going up. It's also known that infections, tumors and other damage to the kidney can result in hypertension. And today, with the aid of new X-ray techniques, doctors are finding that some hypertensives have kidney damage that couldn't have been detected a few years ago.

Thanks to discoveries by researchers such as Dr. Irvine H. Page, recently retired research director of the Cleveland Clinic Foundation, scientists now know a good part of the story of how the kidney raises blood pressure. The kidney, upon detecting a drop in pressure, releases a substance called renin into the blood stream. Renin is quickly converted, through a series of chemical reactions, into another substance called angiotensin. Angiotensin is the most powerful substance known for raising blood pressure; injection of only a few millionths of a gram will send pressure soaring.

One way angiotensin raises blood pressure is by causing constriction of the tiny arteries, the garden hose nozzle effect. But angiotensin has a second, more subtle effect which involves a hormone called aldosterone which is secreted by the tiny adrenal glands that lie atop the kidneys.

Dr. John H. Laragh and his colleagues at Columbia-Presbyterian Medical Center found in the early 1960's that people suffering the malignant or accelerated type of hypertension had an excessive amount of aldosterone circulating in their blood. They then found that angiotensin can trigger the adrenal glands to release aldosterone.

The significance of the findings immediately struck the researchers and has led to the current chemical theory of accelerated hypertension and, some researchers suspect, of the more common types of hypertension.

Aldosterone's main job in the body is to force the kidney to retain salt in blood. In the absence of aldosterone, the kidney will excrete salt in the urine; in its presence, the kidney will hold salt.

Keeping the right concentration of salt in the blood undoubtedly stems from the fact that life first developed in a warm salty primeval sea billions of years ago. If, for some reason, aldosterone prods the kidney to retain more salt than necessary, then the body starts retaining water to dilute it and get the concentration down to normal, which presumably is the same concentration that existed in the primeval sea.

This retention of excess salt and consequently of additional water increases the amount or volume of fluid flowing through the blood system. A greater volume of fluid, like more water being forced into the garden hose, results in higher blood pressure in the arteries.

"Our thesis is that in (accelerated) hypertension something has gone wrong with the kidney's control of salt balance and blood pressure," Dr. Laragh explained some time ago. For some reason, the kidney releases too much renin in the blood thus generating excessive amounts of angiotensin. The angiotensin, in turn, triggers both the constriction of the arteries and the release of aldosterone. The aldosterone raises the level of salt water in the blood, thus boosting blood pressure even more.

If this is correct, then the key to accelerated hypertension would be in finding out why the kidney is releasing too much renin in the first place. In a normal situation, the moment the kidney is "told" by the aldosterone to retain salt, it should shut off the release of renin, but in accelerated hypertension this apparently doesn't happen. Instead, the whole system seems to have gotten out of control.

A host of experiments, mostly in animals, suggest the reason may be some kind of damage to the kidney such as the obstruction of local arteries. This causes a localized drop in blood pressure while leaving the pressure normal in the rest of the body. The kidney's built-in barostat, sensing the drop in pressure, tries to correct it by releasing renin and setting off the whole chemical chain of events. Blood pressure throughout the body that had been normal rises. Meanwhile, the kidney is unable to get its own internal blood pressure up because of the damage and thus continues to release renin. Thus the whole pressure-regulating system gets out of control to create the accelerated-type of hypertension.

If this is the situation in the accelerated kind of high blood pressure, then, perhaps, more subtle variations of it underlie at least some of the cases of so-called essential hypertension, Dr. Laragh and others reason. Maybe, some suggest, instead of the system getting totally out of control, the kidney's barostat is just reset permanently at a high level of pressure.

This theory and the discoveries that led to it are opening up new research avenues. Dr. Laragh and his associates, for instance, have found there may be at least three broad groups of hypertensives, one of which may not be as prone to developing stroke and other complications of hypertension. Using newly developed laboratory techniques they've been measuring the amount of renin in the blood of hypertensives. They've found indications that those with abnormally low amounts of renin in the blood seem to have fewer strokes and heart attacks than those with normal or high amounts of renin, even though they have the same degree of high blood pressure.

These differences in renin levels, as well as similar differences in aldosterone output in hypertensives, suggest to Dr. Laragh that there may be a host of different kinds of essential hypertension. Treatment, he argues, should be tailor-made for each type. In fact, he suggests, some of the more "benign" types of hypertension, such as the low-renin type, may not need immediate drug treatment, a suggestion that has raised considerable controversy.

At the Cleveland Clinic, Dr. F. Merlin Bumpus and his colleagues are in the midst of a search for entirely new types of drugs to treat hypertension. Their tack is to find drugs that interfere with the pressure-raising action of angiotensin. This is an arduous task since they have to know the exact chemical make-up of angiotensin and then create variations of it that would block the natural substance's action. Nevertheless, they've recently come up with some of these angiotensin "analogs" that appear to work in animals.

Drugs already available are effective in lowering high blood pressure. One group of drugs, bearing such trade-names as Diuril and Esidrix, are diuretics. They help control mild hypertension by increasing the excretion of salt and lowering the amount of water in the body or, in other words, reducing the volume of blood. A second broad group of drugs work by blocking the nerve impulses that cause the nerves to constrict the tiny blood vessels, raising pressure. These nerve-blockers bear such trade names as Aldomet, Eutonyl and Ismelin and they include the tranquilizer, reserpine. Often, in moderate and severe hypertension, combinations of drugs are used.

The main drawback to present-day drugs for high blood pressure isn't so much the drugs but the patient. A person with high blood pressure doesn't feel sick, doctors explain. When he takes the drugs and his pressure drops to normal he doesn't feel any relief of pain or any other symptoms; indeed, some people will feel a bit worse because of the drugs. Yet, the drugs have to be taken daily for life. In this situation, a lot of hypertensives will tire of taking the drugs and discontinue them even though their physicians have told them this would likely shorten their lives.

In the near future Americans are likely to see a public health campaign mounted against hypertension that will rival or surpass the campaigns against polio, tuberculosis and, more recently, venereal disease. Federal surveys indicate 15% to 20% of adult Americans suffer high blood pressure, defined as being 160/95 or higher. This multiplies out to between 20 million and 25 million people, making hypertension one of the most—if not the most—prevalent serious ailment in the nation.

Until recently, the evidence implicating hypertension in stroke and heart attack wasn't strong enough to warrant the tremendous expense and effort that would be needed to get more than 20 million people under medical treatment, public health officials explain. But the findings in 1970 by the Veterans Administration, showing the sharp reduction in strokes and heart failure when hypertension is treated changed this. The study showed that the chance of a hypertensive person developing complications such as stroke over a five year period stood at 55% if he was left untreated;

this risk dropped to 18% if the pressure was lowered by drug treatment. And this doesn't include cutting the risk of a heart attack, statistics for which aren't yet available.

With this evidence in hand, the National Heart & Lung Institute, the American Heart Association and others are preparing an attempt to go out and find the 20 million or more hypertensives and get them under treatment.

The task is Herculean. At least 40% of these people don't know they have high blood pressure. "Others who know they have hypertension have either not been told or don't understand the need for long-term antihypertensive therapy," the Inter-Society Commission says.

The first step, under the plan, is to actually go into the streets and begin taking the blood pressures of millions of Americans. Those who show high blood pressure will be asked to either see their own doctor or return to the clinic for additional readings to make sure the pressure wasn't up temporarily. If the diagnosis of hypertension is confirmed then attempts will be made to get the patient under treatment.

The prospect of such a program is causing considerable agonizing in medical and public health circles. Theoretically, tens of millions of Americans will have to be tested. The prospect of putting millions of people on antihypertensive drugs is a bit overwhelming, as are the thoughts about the tremendous numbers of doctors, nurses and technicians that would be required to screen and treat so many people.

As a practical matter, public health officials aren't certain how effective the screening program will be nor how many of the untreated hypertensives uncovered by the program will end up under treatment. As a result, many of the hypertension screening programs now underway are actually pilot efforts.

Despite the magnitude of the hypertension campaign,

many argue it is necessary. "In the long run it should be less expensive to control hypertension than to care for those who become disabled and economically unproductive as a consequence of the disease," claims the Inter-Society Commission.

VI

Obesity: A Lost Cause?

"Obesity is another trait implicated as a significant coronary risk factor. For many years, data have been available from life insurance actuarial studies indicating that overweight persons have an increased risk of dying from coronary and cerebrovascular disease. Risk is a function of degree of overweight."

So says the Inter-Society Commission for Heart Disease Resources in its master plan on how the United States can reduce the toll of coronary artery disease. The commission's solution to obesity is simple: "Caloric intake (should) be adjusted to achieve and maintain optimal weight." In other words, cut down on the calories and lose weight.

Thus, in its 400-page printed report the Inter-Society Commission dismisses in a few paragraphs what medical scientist are finding to be one of the most complex physical and psychological health problems facing Americans. Increasingly, researchers are discovering that for many people obesity may have its roots in the first few months of life and that cutting down on calories isn't such a simple solution.

The commission's view is understandable. Heart specialists generally believe that overweight in itself—at least moderate overweight—isn't an important risk factor. Rather, they explain, overweight people are more prone to develop high blood pressure, high cholesterol levels and diabetes, which are known risk factors for coronary disease.

A moderately overweight person who has normal blood pressure, low cholesterol levels, is free of diabetes and who doesn't smoke has only a slightly higher risk of a heart attack than a person who isn't overweight. (It should be emphasized this applies to *moderate* overweight; extreme overweight is known to be dangerous if for no other reason than overworking of the heart.)

"Correction of obesity is known to be frequently associated with significant control of certain CHD (coronary heart disease) risk factors, e.g., fall in blood pressure of some hypertensive patients, decrease in blood glucose levels in some patients with maturity on-set diabetes," and decline in the amount of fats in the blood, the commission says. Getting down to optimal weight is a "reasonable and safe aspect" of an effort to cut down the risk of a heart attack, the panel claims.

As the commission's report was being serialized in medical journals in 1971, however, Wall Street Journal staff reporter David Brand was exploring a highly disturbing aspect of obesity. Here's what he reported: For decades now, fat people, full of remorse and guilt pangs, have been waddling into their doctors' offices to complain, "I swear, Doc, I've been sticking to that diet you gave me, no fattening stuff at all, and I still gained weight." And for decades now the doctors have sternly accused the miserable fat people of lying.

The doctors may have been wrong. And it seems clear that many fat people were telling the truth all along. A host of new research is revealing a fact that bewilders medical men and that seems certain to dishearten obese people. That fact: Diets and will power are useless prescriptions for those millions of Americans who have been obese since infancy.

Perhaps a third of all fat adults are former fat children. They are doomed. The cure rate for this type of obesity "is worse than the cure rate for cancer of the stomach," says Dr. Hans Neuberg, a New York obesity specialist. "Probably more obese people should stop trying to reduce," says University of Pennsylvania researcher Dr. Albert Stunkard. "It causes more sorrow than anything else."

A spare tire becomes a case of obesity when it adds 15% to 20% to its owner's standard weight. Many Americans do eat their way to such weights but not until middle age. They are the careless ones, and a sensible diet will take their paunches off, just as careful eating thereafter will keep them off. (Heart specialists note this is a vast group of Americans who can reduce the risk of coronary disease by diet.) But many others begin their journey into corpulence during the first few months of life. They were fat in the sandbox and fat all through school. They are fat now and, almost without exception, they will die fat.

Tiny structures called fat cells appear to be the villains that prevent such persons from ever staying thin. Fat cells are located throughout the body, nestled in tissue between the skin and muscles, but they especially accumulate on the abdomen and around such organs as the kidney and heart. Everyone, even the skinniest man, has some fat cells to collect the food eaten, store it and deliver it into the blood stream to be burned as energy. It isn't known if we're all born with the same number of fat cells. But it is known that once a fat cell appears on a person's body it will stay there for that person's lifetime—though the amount of fat any given cell is storing varies from day to day and year to year.

It is also known that the number of these permanent cells

can triple or quadruple in the first few months of life. And there's the rub. The child who waltzes through his Pablum days without gaining any new fat cells will have little trouble staying slim. But the child with an early excess of fat cells is stuck with at least that many cells right to his grave. Furthermore there is something about those excess fat cells, as yet not understood, that makes a normal appetite impossible—that is, that creates a lifetime craving for excess food.

Consequently, even if the person burdened with excess fat cells has, through starvation, lowered his weight to normal, he still carries all those near-empty cells—each one crying out for food, or in some mysterious way telling the body it wants to be fed. Scientists believe this explains why so many once-fat persons who have reduced to thinness promptly regain their spare tires. To compound the problem Dr. Neuberg for one speculates that the person with excess fat cells is in some manner more efficient in using fat—that is, he burns off less fat as energy and puts more into storage than a person with a normal number of fat cells. Thus, the fat person who complains he eats normally but still gains is quite likely telling the truth.

No one yet knows exactly why one child accumulates more fat cells than another, but doctors are beginning to suspect that too much mother love may trigger the problem. It seems clear that the more food a baby eats the more fat cells he develops. And many an American mother, doctors complain, wants her baby to be plump and healthy, so she plies him with goodies.

Of course, it may be that some babies are just more ravenous than others. If so, that would implicate heredity. But a study by the New York City health department found that it's usually the mother, not the baby, that molds the baby's appetite. Rather than listen to their doctor's advice about sensible diets, the surveyed mothers said they paid more attention to advice from relatives, to TV commercials and even to old wives' tales.

However, there's also evidence that the fatter the parents, the fatter their child. A survey of several thousand obese children in the Boston area found that only 7% of the children had parents of normal weight, whereas 80% had obese parents. Scientists lean toward the theory not that obesity is inherited in such cases but that a baby born into a fat family is going to learn fat eating habits—and thus load himself with excess fat cells.

This sort of thing annoys Dr. John Crawford of Massachusetts General Hospital. "This spirit of keeping up with the Joneses by having an infant gobble up formula to produce a better looking growth chart may be leading us astray." And Dr. Neuberg, the New York obesity specialist, declares, "the intestinal tract is the biggest battleground between mother and child in early childhood." Only by encouraging mothers to nourish their children "sensibly and not excessively," he believes, can medical men save millions from a lifetime of obesity.

The stakes are not just cosmetic. A research group at the Medical College of Wisconsin calls obesity a "disease" of "epidemic proportions." It is, they say, probably more critical to national health than malnutrition. From 20% to 25% of Americans who are considered obese run the risk of premature death from a myriad of diseases, including heart disease and diabetes.

Dr. Crawford has found that rats that are lavishly fed from birth do everything sooner than normal rats—including dying. "Everything comes earlier for these luxury animals," he says, "peak running activity, peak body weight and death." Dr. Crawford is reluctant, of course, to say the same thing happens with humans. But the data clearly "suggest to me that longevity is greater in animals that stay lean," he says.

That isn't much help to the person afflicted with a permanent excess of fat cells. For some reason that's still a mystery, such an adult who has been fat since infancy can lose weight only by going on a semi-starvation diet. And he can maintain a slim weight only by sticking for life to a low-calorie diet—a diet that a normal person would lose weight on.

Even when a fat person loses 20, 50, or 100 pounds, all those fat cells remain, like empty balloons waiting to swell up. The way in which infancy-formed fat cells form a base for a lifetime of obesity was discovered by Dr. Jerome Knittle of New York's Mount Sinai School of Medicine and by Dr. Jules Hirsch of Rockefeller University. They redistributed newborn litters of rats among various mothers, giving some mother rats four infants to feed and others up to 22.

The small litters thrived on the abundance of milk. After only a few days they were clearly growing faster than the rats in the larger litters that had to fight for food. In three weeks, Drs. Knittle and Hirsch had a group of fat rats and a group of lean rats. At that point, all the rats were given all the food they could eat. The slim rats stayed slim. The fat rats got fatter.

Some rats were killed, and it was found that fat rats had more fat cells than their lean identical twins. Next, some of the fat rats were starved down to skin and bones and then slaughtered. The researchers found these rats still had a gross excess of fat cells although the cells had shrunk in size and content. Other experimenters have tried to surgically remove these excess fat cells from rats, literally slicing them away. The cells simply grow back again.

Dr. Knittle then turned to humans. In a study of 200 obese

children, he found that there were two-year-olds with double the number of fat cells of a normal adult. (The fat cells were obtained from the children with a special syringe that removed small amounts of tissue from under the skin.)

Dr. Neuberg believes the indestructibility of early-formed fat cells can be explained by a study of anthropology. Such cells, he believes, are a "Stone-age survival mechanism" developed by cavemen who were lucky to find food once a month. Having found food, they would gorge themselves and store the food in their fat cells where it would be slowly released to the body for energy over the weeks of starvation until the next big meal. "Unfortunately, this mechanism is now something like the appendix," he says. "We have no earthly use for it now."

What, then, is there to do for the person stuck with that mechanism? To date, nothing. "Now that we've learned so much about what causes obesity, things are looking pretty bleak," says Dr. Neuberg. Other than intermittent starvation—with the accompanying danger of mental trauma—there is no treatment for taking off the fat and keeping it off. And even starvation may not turn the trick.

Dr. Edgar Gordon of the University of Wisconsin Medical School has another theory. He believes that when the excess fat-cell person goes on a stringent diet he loses protein—that is, muscle tissue—rather than fat. The fat, he says, stays in the fat cells, frustrating even the most rigorous of diets.

Others doubt that, since they have in fact taken the fat off obese patients through starvation. At Philadelphia's Pennsylvania Hospital, Dr. Ted Duncan says he has had great success with a two-week crash diet course. He puts his patients on a diet of black coffee, tea and no-calorie drinks. In this manner, he says, about 1,600 patients have left 11 tons of weight behind them—about 14 pounds per patient, or a pound per patient per day. "It's a drastic step," Dr. Duncan says, "rather like having an appendectomy."

Dr. Duncan says that about 30% of his patients have continued to keep their weight down. He concedes, however, that many of his patients are overweight businessmen who have grown careless as they approach middle age and put on a paunch, or women who have put on excess pounds during pregnancy. Other doctors say it is just such patients for whom reasonable eating habits can take off and keep off pounds. Presumably, the 70% of Dr. Duncan's patients who gain the weight back are persons afflicted with infancy-formed fat cells. In other such crash programs such people lost staggering amounts of weight—and within a short time gained back every pound.

Dr. David Swanson, a Mayo Clinic psychiatrist, tells of a two-year Loyola University experiment he helped conduct with 25 patients, all obese since infancy. In four months, they lost as much as 150 pounds each—more than a pound a day. But within two years, every one of the 25 was obese again.

Some doctors believe this sort of crash dieting for the fat-cell crowd is positively harmful. Dr. Stunkard at the University of Pennsylvania believes such patients will get into a never-ending cycle of losing and regaining weight. Each time weight is added, fat collects along the walls of the arteries. That fat never leaves the arteries—even on subsequent dieting. Thus, the person who gains and loses and gains and loses time and again deposits an additional layer of fat in his arteries with each cycle. The result can be a heart attack.

As yet, doctors have little understanding of the mechanism by which fat cells communicate with the brain's appetite center. They do know, however, that the appetite is mainly controlled by an area of the brain called the hypothalamus. Dr. Crawford, for example, has destroyed the central part of a rat's hypothalamus. The rat ate its way into extreme obesity. It is possible, doctors say, that the human hypothalamus may sometimes go awry—and that the number of infancy-developed fat cells a person carries may have something to do with that dysfunction. That could explain the affliction of numerous obese Americans who are unable to control their appetite. Doctors call them binge eaters.

For such persons, "food has become a form of addiction," says University of Pennsylvania researcher, Dr. Sydnor Pennick. Dr. Swanson of the Mayo Clinic describes binge eating as a sort of frenzy of feeding, often lasting four or five hours at a time. Usually the binge eater will eat in secret and then deny he has eaten to excess. The binger, says Dr. Swanson, does not know when to stop eating.

Others agree. Dr. Pennick says one "extremely obese patient told me that when he's with me he knows when to stop eating only when I tell him. When he's in a restaurant he'll eat until his money is gone. And when he's at home, he'll eat until all the food is gone."

The obese person seems to get sheer pleasure in eating, which has a tranquilizing effect on him, doctors say. Fat people say that's true. "I use food as a tranquilizer all the time," says Shirley Stoler, the 250-pound actress who appeared in the movie, "The Honeymoon Killers." "When life is uncertain or when I'm upset, I eat."

Stuart Byron, a New York free-lance writer, is one obese person who managed to cut his weight from 285 to 161. But to keep it there he had to exist on the edge of starvation. Recently, when Mr. Byron was involved in the production of a movie, he went through "two tense months" and began to eat. He gained 20 pounds, which then had to be taken off slowly and painfully.

A Midwestern newspaperman who is overweight says that sometimes when he is under stress he eats without being aware he is eating. "Once a big story broke 18 minutes before the last edition went to press," he recalls. "In 14 minutes, we had to rip apart the front page and write a lead story on the event. We did it. When it was over, I leaned back in my chair to relax—and discovered that in 14 minutes I had, unknowingly, eaten two large bags of cookies sitting on my desk. Must have been 100 cookies in there. Nothing was left but crumbs all over the desk and my lap and a pair of trousers much tighter than they had been 14 minutes earlier."

Even though doctors are agreed that there is little hope such persons can ever be permanently thin, they still frown on such overindulgence. It's true, they say, that the fat person fat since babyhood will remain fat until death. But if he watches his diet he at least will gain less weight than he would if he simply gorged his way to the grave—and he may even manage to stabilize his current weight.

To some obese person, though, the message is clear: to hell with it. Comedienne Totie Fields is one fat American, who after numerous diets now doesn't "give a damn" about her weight. "I'd rather eat 10 bagels than anything else in the world," she says.

Miss Fields has even decided that being fat is a state of mind. "If people like you they notice you for yourself, not for how much weight you carry. Ed Sullivan once told me, 'Totie, you walk thin.' "

VII

The Psyche and the Heart

Sitting in his office in San Francisco, Dr. Meyer Friedman of Mt. Zion Hospital asks Wall Street Journal reporter James F. Carberry to listen to a tape recording. When he clicks the recorder on a man's voice fills the room. It's startling in its harsh briskness, its impatience in answering a series of questions.

Q. Do you have the feeling that time passes much too quickly for you to accomplish what needs doing each day?

A. I have felt that way constantly for the past several years.

Q. When you play games with your children do you like to win?

A. Certainly. Always.

Dr. Friedman turns off the recorder. "Died about a year ago," he says. "Age 45. Heart attack."

The victim was a successful businessman, married, the father of three. He was time conscious, competitive, a hard charger—a description that would probably fit most successful executives. But Dr. Friedman says the victim belonged to a class of people describable only in superlatives—super time-conscious, ferociously aggressive, frightfully impatient. "These are people whose coat of arms might be a clinched fist wearing a stop watch," says the physician.

Day in, day out, the victim took on a staggering workload, rushed madly from appointment to appointment, bolted his food, mercilessly chewed out laggard subordinates. Compulsively driven to survive in a seemingly menacing world, he gave himself little time for family, friends, leisure. It is men like these that Dr. Friedman and his associate, Dr. Ray H. Rosenman at Mt. Zion Hospital, have been following for more than a decade, comparing what happens to them with the fates of contemporaries who have less frenetic personalities. Their study, covering more than 3,200 California businessmen, has made some startling findings.

Among the supercharged group, which they label Type A Personality, aged 39–49, the death rate from heart attack has been about double that of the others. In the 50–59 age group, where the onset of time normally increases the risk of coronary heart disease regardless of personality, the supercharged group still had a heart attack death rate about 30% higher than the others.

Laymen and heart specialists alike long have felt intuitively that there is a psychological aspect to heart disease and heart attacks, the idea that anger, frustration or some other intense emotion can trigger a heart attack. "Psychosocial tensions related to personal life situations and/or to those inherent in cultural circumstances long have been suspect as factors related to premature coronary heart disease," the Inter-Society Commission says.

Proving that personality and behavoir patterns contribute to coronary disease is difficult since these are extremely tenuous traits to measure. Nevertheless, scientists and physicians are paying increasing attention to the psychological overlay of heart disease. And they are finding that psychological or social stress, if not the basic cause of a heart attack, can at least aggravate or trigger it in people who may have advance stages of coronary disease.

"Clinical experience indicates that emotional crises and unusual fatigue may precipitate acute events (e.g. myocardial infarction, stroke) in persons with pre-existing severe atherosclerotic disease," the Inter-Society Commission notes. This may apply to many other ailments as well as heart attacks.

For example, at the University of Washington, a team headed by psychiatrist Thomas H. Holmes has found that people are more prone to get sick after there has been a major change in their lives. After thousands of interviews, the researchers compiled a list of 40 changes ranked in order of impact on a person: the most wretching change is death of a spouse, followed by divorce, separation and going to jail. The list runs on down to such minor changes as getting a traffic ticket and going on vacation.

The researchers found that more than 80% of the people who had a major life change suffered a major illness within the next two years—and that the more serious the change, the more serious the illness. Dr. Holmes concedes that there is little most people can do about this; their reaction to change, he says, is pretty much built into them. "But what a person can do," says Dr. Holmes, "is to avoid making any other changes that might aggravate the situation. A man whose wife has just died, for example, probably shouldn't try changing jobs or moving to another city for a couple of years."

In an attempt to find out whether a person can literally "die of a broken heart," psychiatrist Dr. William A. Greene and his colleagues at the University of Rochester (N.Y.) Medical Center have been studying the emotional background of people who've suddenly died of heart attacks, that is, people who've died instantaneously or within an hour after they've been rushed into the hospital. Their "study population" is 44,000 industrial workers in Rochester.

In their study, the psychiatrists talked to anyone who was with the patient at the time of his death about the circumstances. In the first two years of the study, the team investigated 54 such sudden deaths among 479 workers who had heart attacks.

"For these patients who have died suddenly, . . . the data available suggests that the majority were depressed and had been for some weeks or months prior to their demise," Dr. Greene says in a report prepared for a recent forum for science reporters held by the American Heart Association.

"Their depression appeared to have been brought on by estrangement, disappointment or separation from a significant person, either a son, a daughter, or other family member," Dr. Greene says. "In a few instances, they were overtaxed or disillusioned in their work. The depression encompassed to varying degrees feelings of sadness, uselessness, being unappreciated and helplessness."

In many of the patients, who had been depressed for a long time, there had been some recent emotional change, a sudden deepening of the depression or development of a situation in which the patient had become angry or anxious, Dr. Greene reports. This indicates, he explains, that the psychological ingredient of sudden death from a heart attack isn't just simply anger, or simply anxiety or depression, but a more complex mix of these emotional states.

The Rochester psychiatrists, at the same time, are looking into another phenomenon, the reasons why many people refuse to call a doctor or an ambulance when they suspect they are having a heart attack. They found, first, that the median "delay time" between when a person first develops symptoms of a heart attack and when he arrives at the hospital was an incredible three and a half hours.

"The majority of patients developing even severe chest pain procrastinate, vacillate, or seemingly dawdle much too long in seeking the excellent technical medical care available in present-day coronary care units," Dr. Greene says. Since this could be one factor behind the fact that 60% of heart attack deaths occur before patients reach the hospital, "we wanted to find out why these damn fools take so long to get to a doctor," he explains.

Among those heart attack victims who waited the longest—and thus took the greatest chances of dying—the researchers describe a person who seems much like the Type A personality described by Drs. Friedman and Rosenman. The people delayed seeking help "because they could not tolerate the helplessness entailed with interruption of on-going activities and being sick," Dr. Greene says. "Most of these patients have been very conscientious in their activities and responsible for important work along with others," he explains.

When the heart attack hits, their main anxiety "is the possibility that they may become disabled and unable to carry on their self-imposed obligations in which they are very much involved and usually over-involved. The prospect of giving up this role and having to become dependent, cared for and relatively passive is extremely threatening, perhaps even more menacing than the prospect of their demise," Dr. Greene believes.

Surprisingly, the psychiatrists found that a person who delayed calling for help for hours after the attack hit the first time, will do the same thing when he's hit by a second heart attack, even though he should have learned better by the second time. In such high risk patients, Dr. Greene suggests physicians talk not only with the patient but with the wife or a friend at work about the problem of calling for help. The Type A person obviously won't ask a stranger for help but he may ask a friend.

Researchers also are finding hints of a correlation between heart disease and the stress of work. The relation may show up statistically because people with the type of personality that is prone to early heart attack may choose the more stressful and demanding occupations.

For example, some years ago, Drs. Henry I. Russek and Burton L. Zohman of New York found that of 100 young coronary patients, 91 suffered from unusual job stress. In a control group of 100 comparable but healthy young men, only 20 had jobs with similar stresses.

The 91 young cardiacs commonly worked 60 hours a week, often in occupations with much frustration, anxiety and discontent. Many of the patients were moonlighting in second jobs.

Another study, this time of the medical profession, showed that heart disease is two or three times more prevalent among family physicians than among dermatologists. The latter speciality has regular working hours and a relatively small amount of stress. Similarly, according to Dr. Russek, stockbrokers have more heart disease than security analysts.

There also are hints of an association between job stress and ailments that add to the risk of developing a heart attack. Air traffic controllers, whose occupation is considered to involve a high degree of prolonged psychological stress, have an unexpectedly high incidence of high blood pressure according to a recent study.

The study was made by Dr. Sidney Cobb, an epidemiologist studying psychological and sociological factors in disease, and Dr. Robert M. Rose, an expert in psychosomatic medicine.

In their study, the two researchers compared the incidence of high blood pressure, peptic ulcers and diabetes in air traffic controllers and in second-class airmen, the pilots who fly commercial aircraft and do the bulk of the flying in the U.S. (First-class airmen are pilots for the big, scheduled airlines while third-class airmen are private, not-for-hire pilots.) The two groups were picked for comparison because they both have to undergo annual physical examination to maintain their licenses and the examinations are carried out by the same groups of physicians. The records of the examination were available from the air surgeon's office of the Federal Aviation Administration.

The researchers found high blood pressure, or hypertension, was four times as common among the air traffic controllers as among the second-class airmen. In addition, the number of new cases of high blood pressure discovered by the annual examination was six times greater among the air traffic controllers than among the pilots. And the incidence was greater among controllers working in centers of high-density air traffic than among controllers in low traffic centers.

Drs. Cobb and Brown, in their report in the Journal of the American Medical Association, said pilots might tend to withdraw from their jobs knowing they couldn't pass the physical or that the examination had weeded out hypertensive pilots at an early stage, thus exaggerating the differences between the two groups. But they said such factors couldn't account for the four-fold higher incidence of hypertension.

As a result of the study, the FAA has other studies under way to try to measure how much stress is encountered on an air controller's job, compared with other types of occupations, and to see if it is a type of job that appeals to people who need to work under psychological stress.

I Think I'm Having a Heart Attack

A person can't do much about changing his personality or how he reacts to stress, of course. But doctors do believe the heart attack-prone personality can do some things to cut down on outside stresses and, particularly to get other risk factors such as smoking, hypertension, and cholesterol levels, under control. For example, an independent petroleum engineer from San Antonio, who suffered a heart attack at age 38, recalls "All my life I worked a 10 to 12 hour day. I operated on Adrenalin, coffee, cigarets and temper." He was also 30 pounds overweight.

Three months after he suffered the attack that left him critically ill for 12 days, he was adjusting to a new regime calling for exercise and controlled diet but excluding "intense business pressures."

By contrast, a Texas cardiologist predicts that one of his patients, a 41-year-old salesman, will be dead within two years. Despite two heart attacks within two years, this man continues to smoke two packs of cigarets a day, remains 30 pounds overweight and shuns exercise.

VIII

When It Happens

If you're going to suffer a heart attack you'd probably be "fortunate" if it happened in Columbus, Ohio. The odds of your surviving would be much better in Columbus than in most parts of the country. David P. Garino, a reporter for The Wall Street Journal, cites the case of Edmund D. Doyle, a partner in the law firm of Porter, Stanley, Platt & Arthur in Columbus. Mr. Doyle was discussing a corporate-reorganization plan with two partners in an 11th-floor office when he felt a pain in his left arm and a tightening in his chest. A partner became alarmed and called the Columbus Fire Department's emergency squad. Within five minutes a three-man paramedic team arrived, took one look at Mr. Doyle and started intravenous treatment and administered oxygen. He was a textbook case of a heart attack victim —sweat on the forehead, a gray, ashen appearance and difficulty with breathing.

The emergency squad placed Mr. Doyle on a stretcher and removed him to an ambulance. Two miles along the way, however, Mr. Doyle's heart stopped. Quickly, a paramedic applied a defibrillator to Mr. Doyle's chest which shocks the heart to restore its normal rhythm. A drug, lidocaine, was administered to prevent erratic heartbeat

71

and thereafter recovery was routine. A half-dozen years ago Mr. Doyle would have been dead.

Such on-the-spot emergency care for heart attack victims saved 202 lives in Seattle over a three-year period, doctors there estimate. And Dr. Richard S. Crampton, director of coronary-care systems at the University of Virginia Medical Center reports that in Charlottesville, the rate for people dying of heart attacks before they could be brought to a hospital was reduced 26% in 1972, largely because of the special ambulance crews' ability to restart stopped hearts.

Despite their potential for reducing heart attack deaths, mobile emergency-care systems are relatively new. Columbus, which set up its unit in 1969, was one of the pioneers. Now over 150 communities, including Jacksonville, Miami, Seattle, Los Angeles, Chicago and New York have similar systems, compared with a mere handful in 1969. A massive regional program is being set up for the Kansas City, Mo., metropolitan area. It will eventually encompass a two-state, eight-county, 110-community area.

Advocates of these systems point to some startling figures: Of the more than one million Americans stricken by heart attacks each year, over half of the victims never reach the hospital alive. The key to saving many lives is to get qualified emergency care quickly to the heart-attack victim, stabilize his condition and then get him to a hospital.

Unfortunately, the national average response time to emergencies is 44 minutes. In some cases, doctors say, the ambulances are nothing more than "horizontal taxis," unequipped to provide medical care. Columbus, operating with four special ambulance units, has trimmed its response time to around five minutes.

In congested areas such as New York City, lifesaving equipment has been installed in many office buildings, including the New York Stock Exchange. And New York's

St. Vincent's Hospital, one of the first in the nation to offer early care to heart-attack victims, restricts itself to a four-square-mile area in the southern part of Manhattan.

These emergency services are provided mainly by fire-department personnel, but police departments, volunteers and private ambulance firms are also used. The paramedics, usually trained by hospitals or medical schools, can provide other emergency care besides aiding heart-attack victims, of course.

In addition to the specially-trained paramedics, a key part of the system is the elaborately equipped ambulance. One of the most sophisticated of such ambulances is the Heartmobile, a prototype vehicle used in the pioneering Columbus system. The Heartmobile has its own electric power supply, refrigerator, water supply and air conditioning. It has an electrocardiogram, oxygen supply, and defibrillator. It also carries a portable electrocardiogram and defibrillator enabling the paramedics to rush to a victim and treat him on-the-spot if he can't be moved. The electrocardiograms can be radioed to the hospital where heart specialists can instruct the paramedics by radio on emergency treatment.

Many once-skeptical doctors are beginning to recognize the value of paramedics. Al Scoles, a battalion fire chief in Columbus, says "We've come a long way. I remember when doctors accused us of practicing medicine without a license when we delivered babies, but then they realized the babies were going to come anyway."

Until recently, efforts to set up early-care systems had little national coordination, but in late 1971 six drug companies formed the Acute Coronary Treatment (ACT) Foundation to promote such systems.

In one instance, a television appearance by ACT Foundation officials prompted a private citizen to press for formation of a mobile coronary-care program in 10 Chicago suburbs. Mrs. Jan Schwettman of Inverness, Ill., who had seen several friends die of heart attacks in their 40s, badgered local politicians and fire departments until a program was established. At one point the fire chief of a Chicago-area village was resuscitated by his own men.

The Kansas City program got its start after a physician's close call with death. In the fall of 1971, Dr. Charles Workman, an orthopedic surgeon, awakened with symptoms of a heart attack. "Then the nightmare that happens in every city began," he recalls. Neither he nor his wife, Myra, a registered nurse, knew how to contact emergency services; after a call to the police an ambulance was finally dispatched and Dr. Workman reached a hospital an hour later.

"I made a promise that if I didn't die, I'd do something to remedy the situation," he says. It was Dr. Workman who pushed the plan for a regional system in Kansas City.

For the half million heart-attack victims who do make it to the hospital each year, the chances for survival have been going up dramatically in recent years. A decade ago, an estimated 35% of heart attack patients who were rushed to the hospital alive subsequently died in the hospital. The most common cause was development of an arrhythmia, an irregular or abnormal heartbeat. Today, in hundreds of hospitals, this death rate among hospitalized heart attack patients has been cut by as much as 50%.

The key to this saving of lives is the coronary care unit, a special ward of four to 12 beds where heart attack victims spend their first day or two. To find out what goes on in one of these space-age wards, reporter William M. Carley visited one when the coronary care unit was just starting to come into its own. His report:

Pip . . . pip . . . pip pip pip pip.

The "pips" come from electronic equipment monitoring the heartbeat of a patient in Boston's Peter Bent Brigham

Hospital. The patient suffered a heart attack only a few hours ago, and the sudden speedup of pips indicates his heart is going into a fatally rapid heart beat.

Hearing the pips, nurses on duty quickly summon doctors. They give the patient an injection of a drug that should make his heart slow down. If the shot doesn't work within a few seconds, the doctors will touch a 1,000-volt electrical charge to the patient's chest in an attempt to shock the heart back into its normal beat.

By alerting doctors to impending complications of the heart attack, particularly the abnormal heart beats, early enough for effective treatment, monitoring equipment is saving the lives of many patients.

At Peter Bent Brigham, for instance, only 17% of 130 heart patients in the coronary care unit died during a 12-month period whereas, in hospitals without such units, the death rate runs between 30% and 40%. In New York, only 21% of some 400 patients in a coronary unit at New York Hospital-Cornell Medical Center suffered fatal complications of heart attack while 32% of the patients in regular accommodations died.

And Dr. Paul Unger, a University of Miami professor, says a study showed the death rate was significantly lower in the coronary unit at Miami Heart Institute, "despite the fact that only the sickest patients were admitted to the coronary unit and despite the fact that patients in ordinary accommodations sometimes were shifted to the coronary unit when they took a turn for the worse."

Behind these dramatic results is ability of the monitoring equipment to detect the abnormal heart beats in time for doctors to correct the heart's rhythm. Even if a person survives his initial heart attack long enough to get to a hospital "he is still in mortal danger," explains a Peter Bent Brigham heart specialist.

I Think I'm Having a Heart Attack

"His initial attack may cause fatal disruption of the electrical signals that control the heart beat," the specialist explains. These electrical signals travel between the upper and lower areas of the heart. If the initial heart attack damages tissue in the heart's narrow electrical pathways, the electrical signals may become erratic. The heart may start beating abnormally fast, or it may grow dangerously slow. Sometimes, some heart muscle fibers will develop their own individual beat completely out of step with other fibers, and the heart goes into a chaotic quivering beat. If allowed to continue, these "arrhythmias" often can lead to stoppage of the heart and death.

In the coronary care unit, the electronic equipment monitors the heart beats by means of two tiny sensors taped to a patient's chest. The sensors detect the bursts of electrical signals that control the beat. The electrical bursts register as "pip" sounds or as a series of sharp peaks on an oscilloscope screen.

Coronary units sometimes also monitor such things as pulse and respiration rates, temperature and blood pressure by means of other sensors taped to a finger, the nose or chest. In many coronary units, a change in the heart beat triggers an alarm buzzer that alerts the hospital staff.

Doctors have effective means of correcting these arrythmias if they can get to the patient in time. In cases where the heart rate is dangerously slow or has stopped, a thin wire is threaded through a vein until it reaches the heart. The wire can carry a small electrical charge into the heart about once a second to force a heart beat. If the beat is stimulated this way for a few hours or days, the heart often seems to mend itself. It starts to send its own electrical signals again, its beat returns to normal, and the artificial "pacemaker" can be removed.

In some cases the heart's electrical system begins a rapid-fire rhythm that can quickly upset the delicate balance of the circulatory system. In this situation, drugs can be used to slow down the racing heart beat. Where drugs won't work, doctors sometimes place two electrodes on the patient's chest and deliver to the heart an electrical charge so large that it momentarily knocks out all the heart's own electrical activity, including the abnormal electrical signals. Somehow, the shock usually restores the heart beat to its normal rhythm.

Doctors until recently used the shock technique very sparingly. If a shock is delivered at a certain vulnerable time in the heart beat, it can make the abnormal heart worse. Recently, however, physicians and engineers have developed electronic monitors that can trigger the shock only at the point in the heart beat cycle that it will be most effective. As a result, this treatment is being used more often.

IX

Limiting the Damage,
a New Theory

The heart attack is a frighteningly simple phenomenon. A segment of one of the tiny coronary arteries, a segment already clogged with fatty deposits, suddenly closes up completely. The part of the heart muscle lying downstream of this blocked artery is deprived of oxygen-rich blood and goes into convulsions. Without oxygen the muscle tissue dies within an hour or so.

There isn't any way to prevent or reverse the death of this muscle tissue. If the damaged area isn't too large, the victim can survive even though part of the heart muscle is no longer functioning.

That, at least, is the way doctors have viewed the heart attack for decades—that the attack is over and done with in an hour or so and about the only thing doctors can do immediately is to relieve the pain and prevent the heart from going into an abnormal rhythm. But this view is now starting to change and, as a result, some new approaches to treating the heart attack victim may be in the offing.

In the last two or three years, medical scientists have developed some new techniques with which they can actually measure the amount of damage inflicted by a heart attack. In the past this could only be done with any accuracy at autopsy. But now the researchers from almost the first hour after an attack, determine whether the damaged area is the size of a dime or a half dollar.

With these techniques, the scientists are finding, much to their surprise, that much of the destruction of heart muscle doesn't occur until many hours or even a few days after the initial attack.

"Just two or three years ago, when a patient came into the hospital, it was assumed he had had his heart attack, that the tissue destruction was completed and that from then on it was a matter of evolving healing," explains Dr. H. Jeremy C. Swan of the Cedars-Sinai Medical Center in Los Angeles and recently president of the American College of Cardiology.

"Today, it's obvious this isn't the case," he says. "Some of the tissue may die quite rapidly, perhaps in the first 30 minutes, but the quantity may not be very great. Other muscle tissue may take hours or days to develop damage."

The implications of this discovery are rather startling. If much of the damage from a heart attack is occurring after the patient is in the hospital, then there's a chance doctors could limit the damage and avoid what otherwise might have become a fatal heart attack.

"Five years ago nobody even thought along these lines, much less acted," Dr. Swan says. Now, however, a host of experiments are under way at major medical centers to see if, indeed, the destruction of heart tissue can be limited.

Early returns hint strongly that it can. One study, for example, suggests that infusions of nitroglycerin in the first few hours after a heart attack can prevent the damage from spreading. Other studies indicate that a careful lowering of high blood pressure could be of vital importance.

The chances of surviving a heart attack once in the hospital are already rising, of course, thanks to the new coronary care units and their ability to detect immediately when the damaged heart develops an abnormal rhythm.

"However, 15% of all patients with myocardial infarction who reach the coronary care unit are still doomed to die," says Dr. Burton E. Sobel, director of the cardiovascular division of the Washington University School of Medicine in St. Louis.

"Death occurs," he explains, "during the acute episode or subsequently and is often associated with signs of 'pump failure,' a condition in which the performance of the heart is so impaired that it can no longer fulfill its basic function of effectively pumping blood. Consequently, blood pressure declines and fluid accumulates in the lung."

It was this mysterious pump-failure type of death that prompted some medical scientists such as Dr. Eugene Braunwald of Harvard Medical School to put forth a theory. They speculated that the pump fails when amount of damage to the heart muscle passes a critical size. It's now thought this failure point is when more than 40% of the lower left chamber is destroyed. It is the lower left chamber that is responsible for pumping oxygenated blood through the body.

In some patients, it's theorized, the damage of the initial attack makes it difficult for the heart to keep an adequate supply of blood flowing through the arteries—particularly the tiny coronary arteries that nourish the heart muscle. Heart muscle tissue surrounding the area of initial damage starts dying for the lack of sufficient oxygen and the area of destruction begins to widen. As additional tissue is destroyed it becomes ever more difficult for the heart to pump adequate blood through the coronaries and a vicious circle develops. Eventually, the tissue destruction spreads beyond the critical point and the pump fails totally and fatally.

Limiting the Damage, a New Theory

If this view is correct, the scientists reasoned, then pump failure could be prevented by either of two methods. One would be to get a new supply of oxygen-rich blood to the threatened area of the heart, an approach that probably would require emergency surgery. The other approach would be to reduce the workload of the heart, thus reducing its need for oxygen to the point where even its impaired blood flow would be sufficient to keep the muscle tissue alive. In this way the vicious circle might be broken and pump failure averted.

To see if this theory is true the researchers would have to be able to measure the initial damage of a heart attack, then watch for hours or days to see if it spreads and if the various treatments could stop it from spreading. Obviously, it's impossible to keep a person lying around for hours or days with his chest open. So the researchers are developing a number of indirect but fairly accurate techniques for measuring and monitoring heart damage.

Dr. Sobel and his colleagues in St. Louis, for example, are capitalizing on the fact that when the cells of the heart muscle are destroyed they release certain chemicals into the blood stream. They've found that the amount of one of these chemicals, called CPK (for creatine phosphokinase) in the blood after a heart attack is a good indicator of how much muscle tissue has been destroyed. More important, with considerable experience under the belt, they can chart the rise and fall of CPK levels in the first few hours after a heart attack and then forecast how much additional damage is likely to occur.

The CPK measures are being used to check the effectiveness of at least one proposed new treatment for certain heart attack victims. These are patients who, in the throes of a heart attack, have high blood pressure. This means the damaged heart has to work harder to pump against the high pressure in the arteries, thus increasing its oxygen demands and threatening to start off the vicious circle leading to pump failure.

The researchers reason that if they can lower the blood pressure by infusing a pressure-lowering drug, they can ease the workload on the heart muscle, reducing its oxygen needs and thus preventing the spread of damage. In the first 15 patients treated this way, the CPK levels in 13 of the patients started dropping considerably earlier than the researchers had forecast. This, they believe, was a sure sign that destruction of the heart muscle had been stopped short of what it might have been.

Dr. Sobel says it is too soon to know whether lowering high blood pressure in these patients will result in saving lives. However, he adds, out of 10 patients with extensive, life-threatening damage to the heart who were treated in this manner only two died. By comparison, out of another group of 10 similar patients who didn't receive the treatment, seven died in the hospital.

In Los Angeles, Drs. Swan and William Ganz are using a different technique. They've developed a long, thin tube—a catheter—with a tiny balloon at its tip. The catheter can be quickly slipped into a blood vessel and pushed up to any of several points near the heart. Flow of the blood against the tiny balloon gives a measure of how forcefully the heart is pumping blood. This, in turn, gives a picture of how well or how poorly the heart is working. With the catheter plus other tests, the researchers can tell whether a patient is in danger of pump failure.

The Los Angeles scientists are now using this approach to see if drugs that dilate or open up the arteries can prevent the spread of damage and pump failure. The larger the artery the less resistance it offers to the flow of blood. Thus, the heart doesn't have to work as hard to pump adequate blood through dilated arteries and its oxygen needs are less, it's reasoned.

In their latest report, Drs. Swan and Kanu Chatterjee and their colleagues say they were able to spot 15 heart attack patients who were almost certain to die of pump failure. All 15 were treated with the dilating drugs and nine of them survived. In another group of 19 similarly treated patients with slightly less damage but still at a high risk of pump failure, 12 survived. In other words, the treatment appears to have cut the risk of pump failure death in these patients to 30% or 40% from 90% to 100%.

Other researchers are using a highly sophisticated version of the electrocardiogram to chart heart attack damage—and they are discovering some unsuspected aspects of the heart attack. The electrocardiogram plots the passage of natural electrical impulses through the heart muscle, impulses that cause it to contract. Where the normal pathways of these impulses are destroyed by a heart attack there will be characteristic squiggles on the electrocardiogram.

Ordinarily, doctors use electrocardiograms that monitor the impulses with only six or 12 wires pasted on the chest. This is sufficient to tell whether the heart has been damaged and roughly where the damage is. But now the researchers are using electrocardiograms with literally dozens of wires pasted to the chest above the heart.

These new electrocardiograms can provide a detailed map of the heart showing the exact location of the damaged area and how extensive it is. They can be used to monitor the heart hour by hour or day by day to see if the damage is spreading and if a particular treatment is limiting or even reversing the spread of destruction.

At Johns Hopkins University medical school in Baltimore, a team of researchers, for instance, is using an electrocardiogram with 48 wires pasted in closely placed rows on the chest. They are evaluating the infusion of nitroglycerin in patients in the first few hours after a heart attack. Nitroglycerin is known to dilate the coronary arteries. So it's hoped the drug will either decrease the workload on the heart or, by opening up the coronaries, will boost the flow of oxygen-rich blood to the heart tissues surrounding the damaged area, keeping them alive.

In the first several patients, the nitroglycerin appeared to work. The electrocardiogram maps showed the work of the left pumping chamber improved markedly and, indeed, the size of the oxygen-starved area actually shrank.

The Johns Hopkins researchers also have uncovered an unsuspected peril to heart attack patients with their electrocardiogram mapping. They made such maps daily on 14 patients beginning on the day they were brought into the hospital. In at least 12 of these patients they discovered that the damaged area suddenly began widening about the fifth or sixth day after the heart attack.

By the fifth or sixth day the patients usually have been moved out of the coronary care ward and into the regular room and aren't being as closely watched as initially. Thus, such a belated extension or continuation of the heart attack wouldn't be noticed. Since doctors didn't know this extension of the heart attack could happen, patients' complaints of chest pains were usually ascribed to something else.

As a result of this discovery, the Johns Hopkins researchers suggest that the new damage-limiting treatments might be useful for several days after the heart attack, not just in the first several hours. The electrocardiogram mapping might also be useful in ferreting out those patients who need emergency surgery to implant new blood vessels to the heart and bring in a fresh source of oxygenated blood.

In the near future, mapping of the damage from a heart

attack might be greatly simplified. Several researchers have found that radioactive potassium injected into a patient will migrate to the heart. The potassium will be picked up by healthy heart muscle but won't be taken up by heart muscle deprived of blood by the heart attack, explains Dr. Bertram Pitt at Johns Hopkins.

A radiation detector can scan the chest after an injection of radioactive potassium and record quite accurately which part of the heart muscle is receiving blood and which isn't.

At the University of Chicago, other researchers have found that radioactive ammonia is even faster and perhaps better than potassium for such use. Unfortunately, ammonia loses its radioactivity fairly rapidly—in a matter of hours —after it is made radioactive in a nuclear reactor. Thus, it can be used only in hospitals that have a nuclear reactor nearby.

Meanwhile, cardiologists are anxiously awaiting the test results of another potentially new treatment that might save lives in the first few hours after a heart attack: an unusual chemical that can dissolve blood clots.

The chemical is called urokinase and is an enzyme found in minute quantities in human urine. It is being produced for experimental use by Abbott Laboratories and Sterling Drug Co. from urine collected at several military installations.

The testing of urokinase is being watched closely by the medical profession because blood clots are a major cause of death in the U.S. Many—but not all—heart attacks are thought to be due to blood clots finally plugging up a coronary artery already clogged by atherosclerosis. In addition, there are thousands of deaths every year due to blood clots blocking arteries in the lungs. It long has been a dream of physicians to find a way to get rid of these clots before they can inflict their oft-fatal damage.

I Think I'm Having a Heart Attack

The interest in urokinase has been intense ever since researchers announced, in 1970, the results of its use in a carefully controlled clinical trial involving 160 persons suffering the lung clots or pulmonary embolisms, as they're called. The clinical trial "represents the first time the clot-dissolving potential of any agent ever has been established unequivocally in man," Dr. Sol Sherry, the Temple University scientist who headed the trial, told the American Heart Association at the time.

Laboratory tests indicated a few years ago that urokinase probably had the ability to dissolve clots in humans. When it came time to test it in humans, researchers wanted to avoid a pitfall that has plagued other chemicals thought to have clot-dissolving activity.

In the late 1950's two clot dissolvers were marketed with considerable fanfare. One was quickly taken off the market because side effects were more severe than early tests indicated. The second is still available but isn't widely used because the clinical trials failed to prove that the disappearance of the clot was due to the chemical and not to the body's natural clot-dissolving ability.

With urokinase, the researchers decided to test it with one of the most carefully planned clinical trials in modern medicine so there would, in the end, be no doubt about whether it is effective or not. Although they wanted to try urokinase in heart attacks, they picked the pulmonary embolism as the first clot disorder to attack. This is because there are methods of using X-rays and radioactive tracers, as well as other tests, that can clearly show the size and location of the clot in the lungs before and after use of urokinase. Such methods are being developed for heart attacks.

Pulmonary embolism is a leading cause of death in hospitals. It occurs when a clot breaks loose from the walls of a vein, usually veins in the legs. The blood stream quickly carries the clot up the major vein, through the chambers on the right side of the heart and into the lungs. Since, in the lungs, the blood is moving through increasingly smaller arteries, the clot eventually lodges in an artery. If the clot is large enough and blocks off a large artery, the results can be fatal.

If the pulmonary embolus (an embolus is a moving clot) is large and dangerous enough, an emergency operation can be performed to remove it. Otherwise, the principal treatment is to administer drugs called anticoagulants to prevent new clots from being formed and giving the body time enough to get rid of the clot on its own.

The first clinical trial of urokinase was carried out simultaneously at several different medical centers and was funded by the National Heart and Lung Institute. All the centers used exactly the same detailed plan and treatments. Patients in whom tests clearly showed a blood clot existed were told of the trial and its purpose and asked if they wanted to volunteer. Those who did were then randomly assigned to receive either a 12-hour infusion of urokinase or conventional treatment with an anticoagulant. After treatment by either method, tests were again conducted to find out what happened to the clot.

A total of 160 patients volunteered, with 82 being assigned to the urokinase treatment and 78 to conventional anticoagulant treatment. The tests, the researchers say, clearly showed that in the patients treated with urokinase the clot either disappeared or shrank in size far quicker than in the other patients and that blood circulation in the lungs reverted towards normal sooner.

In addition, 11 of the urokinase-treated patients had massive clots that might normally have been operated on. Only two of these patients died, a death rate that, the researchers say, is "strikingly lower" than the death rate among patients undergoing emergency surgery for pulmonary embolisms.

The clinical trial was aimed only at testing whether urokinase could dissolve a clot. It still isn't known if it will reduce deaths from pulmonary clots. In the trial, 7% of the urokinase-treated patients did die later compared with 9% in the anticoagulant group. In such a small number of people this isn't a statistically significant difference; it would take a trial of 20 to 40 times as many patients to determine if the chemical can significantly reduce the death rate.

A second clinical trial is under way. In the first trial urokinase was infused in the patient for only a 12-hour period. In the second trial a 24-hour infusion will be tried. In addition, a second, older chemical thought to be a clot dissolver will be tested and compared with urokinase.

Meanwhile, plans are being made to try the clot dissolving chemicals in heart attacks.

X

Coronary Cinema

Movies that will never win Academy Awards or mesmerize viewers of the late, late show are becoming a significant weapon against heart disease.

The movies are the product of a relatively new diagnostic technique that allows medical specialists to see and photograph with the aid of X rays, the vital coronary arteries, the tiny vessels that furnish life-sustaining blood to the heart muscle. The technique enables doctors to judge how badly arteries may be clogged with the fatty deposits of atherosclerosis and even to determine the severity of the clogging before a heart attack occurs. It thus helps them determine how far they must go in using surgery or drugs to prevent disabling heart damage or life-threatening heart attacks.

Equally important, the technique has spotted hundreds of instances where older, less accurate diagnostic methods had led doctors to erroneously diagnose heart disease in patients. Were it not for the new technique, say physicians, these patients might have gone through life believeing they had a "bum ticker" and afraid to climb two flights of stairs or play a game of tennis.

The X-ray movies are proving most useful in angina pectoris, that painful feeling of tightness in the chest, usually occurring after exertion, emotional stress, eating a heavy meal or other conditions that place an extra demand on the heart. The pain indicates the coronaries have become so narrowed the heart muscle can't get enough blood to meet the extra demand.

Angina pain is as sure a symptom of coronary atherosclerosis as is the heart attack, the only difference being its lack of suddenness. Left untreated, the pain gradually becomes more and more frequent upon less and less exertion and can reach the point of totally disabling a person. It is in confirming the diagnosis of angina and mapping out its treatment that the coronary artery movies are being widely used.

The technique, perfected by Dr. F. Mason Sones Jr. of the Cleveland Clinic, bears the formidable name of "selective cine coronary arteriography," meaning simply that it selects the coronary arteries alone for motion picture X-ray photography. Basically, it's a method to fill the coronary arteries with a fluid that makes these vessels visible on fluoroscopes and X-ray film. Blood vessels ordinarily are invisible when the body is X-rayed and, until now, the only way to look at the coronary arteries was through major surgery.

Coronary arteriography works like this: The conscious patient lies on a table beneath an X-ray machine equipped with an "image amplifier," a device that brightens the X-ray image of the patient to permit high speed motion pictures to be made. A small incision is made in the right arm or leg under local anesthesia and an artery is opened. A thin plastic tube called a catheter is inserted into the artery and pushed carefully up inside the artery into the chest until it reaches the beginning of the main artery, the aorta, that leads off the top of the heart.

Near this point on the main artery are two small openings leading to the coronary arteries; one leads to the arterial

90

network serving the right side of the heart, the other into the left. As specialists watch the image amplifier, the tip of the tube is guided carefully into one of these coronary artery openings.

The image amplifier screen now shows shadowy images of bones and the sharp, black image of the catheter tube seemingly resting in the middle of nothing; the heart, blood vessels and other soft tissues are all but invisible.

Then doctors quickly inject into the tube a fluid which is opaque to X-rays and appears black on the image screen. The fluid shoots into the coronary artery and, as it fills, a black, tree-like web suddenly appears on the screen, moving back and forth as the heart contracts and expands. In a few seconds the fluid is washed away by the flowing blood and its image disappears.

Meanwhile, a movie or a television camera is recording the events on the image screen. Both coronary arteries are made opaque, usually several times, with the patient in a different position each time to allow an all-round view of the coronary network.

By closely studying these movies later, specialists can spot areas where there is a sudden narrowing of the flow of the black fluid, indicating an obstruction such as a fatty deposit in the artery. They also can detect points where the flow of the fluid suddenly stops because of complete blockage of the artery.

With present equipment, says Dr. Sones, arterial branches as small as five-thousandths of an inch in diameter can be seen. The technique, he adds, also can detect as little as a 10% narrowing of the main coronary artery; painful symptoms usually don't develop until an artery is nearly half closed.

Insertion of the catheter, says Dr. Sones, who speaks from personal experience, is relatively painless because the arteries through which it passes have no sensory nerves. "A patient sometimes will get irritated with all of our fussing around and his artery will clamp down on the catheter," he notes. This will cause an aching discomfort in the arm or leg. It requires 45 minutes to an hour to get a complete view of the coronary arteries.

The idea of injecting X-ray-opaque fluid into the blood vessels so they can be seen on X-ray fluoroscopes and films dates back three to four decades. At least since World War II doctors have developed the method to examine such things as obstructions in the kidney's blood vessels or the condition of the valves in the heart. But Dr. Sones is credited with being the first to be able to single out the tiny coronary arteries for visualization and motion picture photography. He first performed it on dogs between 1956 and 1958 and on the first human in the latter year.

The Cleveland group since then has accumulated by far the greatest experience with coronary arteriography. By 1964 it had used it on more than 3,300 persons referred to the clinic from all over the U.S. Today, it is available in almost all major medical centers.

"Its primary use is in evaluating patients where the diagnosis (of coronary atherosclerosis) isn't clear-cut or in patients where certain types of surgery are contemplated," explains a cardiovascular specialist at the Hahnemann Medical College and Hospital in Philadelphia, one of the centers to begin using the technique in the early 1960's.

Traditionally, doctors evaluating chest pains rely on several indirect methods. Most make the diagnosis of coronary disease by noting such tip-offs as whether pain occurs during exertion and whether it stops when artery-dilating drugs such as nitroglycerin are given. Electrocardiograms also are valuable. Abnormalities in the electrical activity of the heart, as traced out by the electrocardiogram, can indicate some part of the muscle isn't working properly, possibly because of an inadequate blood supply.

Such techniques in many people leave little doubt that the chest pain is true angina pectoris caused by coronary disease. But in others the diagnosis isn't always certain. Electrocardiograms can be misinterpreted since, for example, diseased heart valves can produce abnormalities. And chest pain symptoms described by the patient often aren't objective. One physician's handbook, the Merck Manual, notes that pain due to coronary artery disease "may be called more appropriately a feeling of oppression or distress, and is usually described as squeezing, crushing or viselike, rather than sharp or knifelike." If a patient has a preconceived notion that his chest pain is due to heart disease, he may unwittingly mislead the doctor who's trying to extract an accurate description of the pain.

Small wonder, then, that inaccurate diagnoses appear common in light of the revelations of coronary arteriography. In the mid-1960's an analysis of 1,000 patients who underwent coronary arteriography at the Cleveland Clinic found that 366—more than one out of three—had relatively normal coronary arteries as seen by the technique. Yet all had been diagnosed earlier by older methods as probably suffering from coronary artery disease.

"A large number of these people actually were suffering neuromuscular chest pains," Dr. Sones recalled at the time. "Others had inflammation of the esophagus, a few had bouts of pleurisy and some were simply looking for some condition for which they could collect insurance." Yet the lives of many of these people were being dominated by the belief they had coronary disease.

One of the more distressing cases was that of a woman who, for six years, had suffered "terrible heart pains." Two heart operations were unsuccessful. Her thyroid gland was

93

then destroyed by radiation in the hope this would lower her body's metabolism and thus reduce the demand on the heart. Arteriography later showed her coronary arteries to be normal. Doctors then decided her pains were psychologically caused and all the previous treatment had been unnecessary.

Even when the diagnosis of coronary artery disease is certain, arteriography can help physicians determine whether surgery would be useful. For example, if only certain sections of an artery are plugged, the patient might be helped by an operation in which the chest is opened and surgeons clean out the artery with an instrument, an operation called an endarterectomy. The X-ray movie, by showing the exact location of the obstruction, takes much of the guesswork out of deciding whether a patient is a candidate for this type of operation.

More important, it is fast becoming a prerequisite for deciding whether a patient can be helped by implanting new blood vessels to the heart muscle to bring in a new blood supply. This type of surgery, called the coronary by-pass, is rapidly becoming the most common type of heart surgery in the nation. The X-ray movies can not only help pick out potential patients but permits the surgeons to map out the surgery ahead of time.

In the months following a heart attack, coronary arteriography can reveal how well the heart has been able to recover and develop new blood vessels that skirt around the obstructed artery that caused the heart attack. It also can reveal whether a patient being considered for such open heart surgery as valve replacement might also have coronary disease that would make him a poor surgical risk.

Proponents of coronary arteriography claim it is both safe and accurate. Of the first 3,300 patients undergoing the procedure at the Cleveland Clinic there were only four cases in which arteriography showed normal coronary arteries in persons who subsequently were proven to have coronary atherosclerosis.

"It's too early to tell whether coronary arteriography will be used routinely for diagnosing angina," says one heart specialist. Adds another, "Diagnosis of typical angina by present methods is pretty straightforward." Most cardiologists, even those with large practices, may run across only one or two patients a week in whom arteriography would be useful, he explains, and these could be referred to major medical centers. This, he believes, would be better than trying to introduce the technique into every community hospital in the nation, which would be a rather expensive undertaking considering the equipment costs $100,000 or so.

However, says a Philadelphia cardiologist, "a lot of doctors who have had no experience with arteriography are still reluctant to have it done (on their patients). I think that, as more doctors become aware it is a benign (safe) procedure, you'll see arteriography being done more and more."

XI

By-Passing the Coronaries

By normal reckoning, the 52-year-old mechanic's case should have been written off as hopeless. For years, his coronary arteries had been clogging up until the blood flow to the heart muscle had been slowed to a trickle. He had suffered six heart attacks and the inadequately nourished lower left chamber of the heart was starting to fail. The man was gulping down 120 nitroglycerin tablets a day trying to ease the attacks of chest pain caused by the diminishing flow of blood.

Instead of preparing for his last days, though, the ailing mechanic elected in 1962 to have an operation at Montreal's big Royal Victorian Hospital. There, for more than two hours, chief surgeon Dr. Arthur M. Vineberg and his colleagues worked delicately in the man's open chest. Their goal: To bring the heart muscle a new blood supply partly by borrowing blood vessels from other parts of the body and grafting them to the heart.

The success of their efforts was evident years later. The man was back at work full time, his need for nitroglycerin had disappeared and his heart was showing signs of recovering from near failure.

The Canadian mechanic's experience is one of the early

episodes in the story of a type of surgery that has suddenly blossomed into the most common open-heart surgery done in the nation. It is surgery to add new blood vessels to the heart muscle to by-pass the disease-ridden coronary arteries. Although versions of it date back almost two decades—to pioneering work by Montreal's Dr. Vineberg—this type of surgery has jumped from a few score operations in 1967 to more than 40,000 in 1973, and its use is growing at the rate of 20% to 25% annually.

Behind this almost unprecedented popularity of the new operations is the fact the surgery relieves the disabling pain of angina pectoris. It can't be used in all patients suffering this symptom of coronary disease—and it isn't successful in all patients where it is tried. But when the surgery works, the results are often dramatic. Doctors can cite case after case of people—from executives to housewives and even athletes—returning to near-normal lives after months or years of crippling chest pain.

The explosion in the use of by-pass surgery, however, is also stirring major concern and even controversy among heart specialists. They are worrying that too many surgeons, either out of eagerness or from intense pressure from patients, are attempting the new surgery when they shouldn't. The result, they fear, is that by-pass operations are being carried out on patients in whom the risks of the surgery outweigh its potential benefits. Indeed, many specialists claim, it isn't even clear yet exactly what kind of heart patient should have the surgery. It may be, they explain, that many patients who could easily be treated with medications are unnecessarily going under the knife.

And, perhaps the most important concern of all, the surgeons themselves aren't yet sure whether the operations prolong life—and they won't know until some carefully planned controlled trials of the surgery are completed in the late 1970's. Should it be proven the surgery prevents an early death from coronary disease, as well as relieves the pain of angina, the operations would be a major advance. Otherwise, use of the surgery may be limited to persons who are so crippled by the angina its relief alone would be worth the risk of an operation.

The new surgery isn't an overnight phenomenon. As early as 1946, Montreal's Dr. Vineberg put forth the idea that since angina pectoris was due to a badly clogged coronary artery failing to deliver enough blood to a part of the heart it might be possible to relieve it by bringing in a new source of blood. Specifically, Dr. Vineberg would detach one end of an artery from the chest muscle behind the breast bone and graft it to the front lower left side of the heart muscle, an area frequently stricken by coronary disease. The chest muscle doesn't suffer since it has a plentiful supply of arteries. Within a few months, if all goes well, the end of the artery implanted to the heart has established itself and is providing the muscle with a new supply of blood.

Dr. Vineberg, from the early years on, was convinced the internal mammary artery implant, as the operation is called, worked. But for years there was considerable skepticism among other surgeons about whether the implanted artery remained open and provided blood to the heart muscle. The relief of angina pain alone wasn't sufficient evidence the operation worked, they argued. Too often, they noted, patients diagnosed as having angina (this was before the advent of coronary arteriography) would improve apparently for psychological reasons. In one experiment, later to become highly controversial on ethical grounds, patients who received a sham operation for angina showed as much improvement as patients who underwent the real surgery, in this case an operation that was subsequently discarded.

However, in 1961 the skepticism over the Vineberg operation suddenly disappeared. This was after Dr. F. Mason Sones in Cleveland used his then-new coronary arteriography to examine a car salesman who had been operated on by Dr. Vineberg seven years earlier. Dr. Sones found that blood was actually flowing through the implanted artery to the man's heart.

On the basis of such evidence use of the Vineberg operation began to spread and coronary arteriography repeatedly confirmed it worked. At the Cleveland Clinic, for instance, surgeon Dr. Donald Effler and his colleagues by 1966 had performed more than 270 such artery implants. Of 68 of these patients in whom they checked the results with arteriography only in seven had the implanted artery failed to remain open. The surgery carried its risks, of course; the Cleveland surgeons reported an operative mortality of 3%.

Cardiovascular surgeons around the nation began attempting to improve the surgery, including Dr. Vineberg himself. His initial surgery involved implanting only the left side of the heart muscle with the left internal mammary artery. But he quickly added other procedures. One is to take a piece of fatty tissue from the abdomen and transplant it to the top of the heart. The tissue, called omentum, is richly laced with blood vessels that quickly attach themselves to the heart opening up new channels between the disease-free arteries at the top of the heart and the blood-starved areas. He also began implanting the right internal mammary artery to the right side of the heart.

In the artery implants pioneered by Dr. Vineberg it requires several weeks, at least, for the new arteries to attach themselves permanently to the heart muscle. In their search for quicker, easier operations to bring in new blood supplies to the heart muscle surgeons such as those at the Cleveland Clinic perfected the operation that is now the most common open heart surgery done in the nation.

In this newer version, a large vein is removed from the leg

(which the leg can easily spare). One end of the vein is then attached to the aorta, the giant artery leading out of the top of the heart. Surgeons, having located the clogged segment of the coronary artery with arteriography, then attach the other end of the vein to a spot on the coronary below the clogged section. In effect, they lay a pipeline around the obstruction in the coronary that is causing the angina.

The new operation is far more versatile than the Vineberg operation since surgeons can pipe new blood from the aorta to almost any part of the heart. Because coronary disease often afflicts several segments of the coronary arteries, most patients receive at least two such by-pass vein grafts and some have received as many as six, all during the same operation.

By carefully picking out the patients who are most likely to benefit from the vein by-pass operations, surgeons around the country are claiming 80% to 90% success in relieving the angina chest pain. About a fifth of the time a grafted vein will close up within a year or so after surgery but since most patients have one or two other grafted veins still open and carrying blood, this isn't thought to be a major problem. The operation carries about a 1.5% to 3% operative mortality, depending on the medical center.

Heart surgeons vary in their enthusiasm for the vein by-pass grafts. Some of its strongest boosters believe it could be done even in the mildest cases of angina if the arteriography shows that the coronaries are badly clogged. Others recommend the surgery only if the person is severely disabled and all other treatment fails. Most, however, agree that a person with moderate to severe angina pain, who hasn't yet had a heart attack and who isn't getting much relief from drugs such as nitroglycerine is a good candidate for the by-pass operation.

Jack March, a 53-year-old tennis pro at the Shaker Racket

Club near Cleveland, for instance, told Jonathan Spivak of the Wall Street Journal his story in the fall of 1972. His angina pain had become so intolerable it not only affected his tennis playing but finally made it painful even to climb a flight of stairs. After the by-pass surgery, he not only was back on the court but entering tournaments. "I'm playing twice as well as before the operation," he said.

But with the number of by-pass operations zooming to almost 40,000 a year in 1973, Mr. Spivak also found considerable concern among heart specialists. "Skeptics fear it's being promoted too hard by enthusiastic surgeons and embraced too eagerly by desperate patients," he reported. "They worry that the operation will be performed unnecessarily at hospitals that are inadequately prepared. The doubters are concerned, too, that the demands of by-pass surgery are straining the nation's blood banks and encouraging the establishment of too many open-heart centers, diverting scarce medical resources from other pressing needs."

As one heart specialist put it at the time: "A lot of smaller institutions or institutions with no previous background in cardiac surgery and without trained personnel to take care of people are starting or already doing the operation. Inevitably, they are going to carry a higher mortality rate . . . It will disenchant many cardiologists because they will see the results in patients who are improperly selected or die on the altar of the ego of the institution and boards of trustees who want to have an open-heart surgery unit."

While the by-pass surgery unquestionably relieves angina pain, it is far too early to know whether it prolongs life. A study at the Cleveland Clinic, which has had the most lengthy experience with the by-pass surgery, hints that it does, at least initially.

But some heart specialists say there are still unanswered

questions about the operation. One major unknown is whether a person after the operation is at a higher or lower risk of having a heart attack, partly because of the mechanics of the by-pass. Surgeons are finding that when the newly grafted vein shunts blood around the diseased "native" artery, the native artery might close up completely just for the lack of blood pressure. This raises the question of what happens if the grafted vessel, itself, closes up later on and there aren't any native arteries left that could take over even partially.

Surgeons also debate whether the operation causes other native arteries "downstream" from the graft to close up more frequently than they would otherwise. If so, the operation would be increasing the risk of a heart attack in the months and years following the surgery.

To answer such questions hundreds of heart patients who have been referred to any of 10 major medical centers are being asked to participate in a controlled study of the by-pass surgery. Those who agree are being randomly divided into two groups, one of which will undergo the by-pass surgery while the other remains under conventional treatment. The patients, of course, are free to withdraw any time they or their doctors have a change of mind; a person on conventional treatment can withdraw if he or his physician decides he would benefit from the by-pass surgery, for instance.

Two types of heart patients will be prohibited from volunteering for the experiment. One type will be those who clearly need the by-pass surgery because their chest pains are so severe they are disabled. The other type is the patient whose chest pains are mild or absent but whose heart is so badly damaged by coronary disease that the surgery would be too risky.

Only those patients who are troubled by moderate chest

pain but in whom it isn't clear the surgery would be of help will be accepted for the study. The researchers will then closely watch the two groups of these patients to see whether those with the surgery have fewer heart attacks and deaths than the non-operated group. The hoped-for life-prolonging benefits of the by-pass surgery may become clear by 1978 or 1979.

XII

The Surgeon

For a growing number of Americans, the thoracic surgeon is becoming an almost mystical figure. It is the thoracic surgeon who performs open-heart surgery, whether it be for a coronary by-pass operation, replacement of a damaged heart valve or transplantation of a new heart. For a short time, he literally holds the patient's heart—and life—in his hands. To get a better understanding of who he is and what he does, Wall Street Journal reporter Richard D. James spent some time with a thoracic surgeon, in and out of the operating room. His 1969 report, which follows, is an excellent study and profile that stands as one of the most informative and insightful on the subject.

A visit to green-tiled operating room No. 2 at Billings Hospital in Chicago creates a fleeting impression of being thrust into the cockpit of a spaceship. Electronic equipment studded with dials and switches stands everywhere. Hanging from the ceiling is a large oscilloscope resembling a television set. Jagged yellow blips of light move across the amber screen. Cables and oxygen hoses are strewn across the floor.

On the operating table, almost covered by green surgical drapes, is a short, balding man of 62. His chest, tinted brown with antiseptic, is exposed to the intense light of fixtures hanging above the table. A 12-inch incision has split open his chest, and the beating heart is visible.

The room, kept slightly chilly for the comfort of surgical personnel, isn't crowded, but there are 16 medical specialists present—the team for open-heart surgery. Standing at the center of the group is Dr. Charles Frederick Kittle, the red-haired, six-foot-four-inch chief cardiac surgeon. With swift, deft movements, he lifts the heart and cuts a four-inch incision in it.

The world of heart surgery has been much in the spotlight recently, due to numerous and dramatic heart transplants. To Dr. Kittle, the dramatic is commonplace. This operation, in which he is replacing one of the heart's four valves, is one of the approximately 1,000 occasions he has performed open-heart surgery, so called because the heart actually is opened while its functions are taken over by a heart-lung machine.

In this same room, on Christmas Day, Dr. Kittle performed the world's 102nd—and Chicago's first—heart transplant operation. The recipient was an eight-day-old boy, the youngest patient yet to undergo such surgery. But the operation failed. The heart, taken from a two-day-old boy, wouldn't continue beating on its own. A pathology report hasn't disclosed why.

Dr. Kittle, 47 years old, is a foremost practitioner among medical pioneers pressing the surgical battle against heart disease, the nation's No. 1 killer. Since 1966 he has been professor of surgery and chief of the section of thoracic and cardiovascular surgery at the University of Chicago's Pritzker school of medicine, of which Billings is a part. The nation's 500 or so heart surgeons constitute an elite among the 25,000 surgeons in the U.S., partly because of the drama of their work, partly for its sheer difficulty and delicacy.

More heart patients die on the operating table than in other forms of surgery. In most cases, the operations are longer and more complicated, the equipment more sophisticated and the operating teams more complex. For the surgeon, the emotional and physical stress is immense. "About the only situation I can really imagine it similar to is a soldier in the front lines of war," says Dr. Kittle, without pomposity.

But if the pressures are large, so is the compensation. A heart surgeon may charge between $1,000 and $3,000 for an open-heart operation, and it's not unusual for heart surgeons in private practice to gross more than $100,000 a year. Dr. Kittle is paid a straight salary by the university, running between $40,000 and $50,000 a year. He receives no fees from patients.

He could make more if he set up his own practice, but Dr. Kittle believes that a surgeon has a responsibility to pass on his knowledge to the next generation of practitioners. Thus, he teaches as well as operates. "It's sort of like sowing the seed rather than going out and reaping all the harvest," he says.

Watching Dr. Kittle replace a heart valve offers a closer look at the existence of the heart surgeon. With this particular patient, rheumatic fever and subsequent infections have scarred a valve and partially destroyed it, causing blood to back up in the man's lungs. Climbing stairs, or simply walking, leaves him breathless. Without surgery, he would be an invalid and probably die within two or three years. There is a 15% chance of death from the operation. But a successful operation may mean an end to shortness of breath and added years of useful life.

Cardiac surgery is a relatively young specialty. Most of the advances have come since World War II. Most spectacular is the heart transplant technique, but a number of other operations have been devised in recent years. Replacement of valves was tried first about 10 years ago, several years after the advent of the heart-lung machine.

The usual procedure is to replace the defective valve with an artificial one made of plastic and steel, but in this case Dr. Kittle is using a homograft—a transplanted valve from the heart of a dead person. Such valves can be frozen and stored indefinitely, and there is no problem of rejection, as in the transplant of an entire heart. Dr. Kittle believes valve transplants result in fewer complications, such as potentially fatal blood clots, than do artificial valves.

Dr. Kittle usually performs three or four heart operations a week and an equal number of lung operations. On this day he arrives at about 8 A.M., as usual, at his office on the fifth floor of Billings, one of seven hospitals in the 675-bed university health center.

The surgery already has begun without Dr. Kittle. At 7 A.M. the patient had been brought up to the operating theater. Scrubbing and other preparations were carried out, and he was put under anesthesia. Now the senior resident surgeon, 30-year-old Dr. Bernard Mizock, is opening the chest cavity.

Dr. Kittle slips into a white, knee-length coat and heads for the operating suite on the sixth floor. First stop is the dressing room, where he changes into green surgical garb. At 8:25, he is in an anteroom off the operating room, where he scrubs for 10 minutes, chatting calmly with the anesthesiologist, Egyptian-born Dr. Adel A. El-Etr. He displays no tension. "I find the atmosphere of the operating room stimulating, but also relaxing," Dr. Kittle says. "I suppose this is from the number of years I've been in it. It's so familiar and comfortable. If I'm feeling out of sorts at all or worried about something, I think the best thing is to go operate. It's comforting."

He was not always so confident. Dr. Kittle recalls his first operation, as a 24-year-old intern in 1945. "It was an appendectomy," he says. "There were no problems as far as the patient was concerned, but it seemed to take a long time and I was a little bit shaky. There's a big difference between helping somebody and picking up the knife and making the incision yourself. I was relieved and happy when it was over."

Now he doesn't worry, and he tries to instill an equal confidence in his associates. "I tell our residents the operating room is no place to worry about whether they can do an operation. It's just like a concert pianist getting up on stage and thinking, 'Gee, I wish I'd done those scales a little bit more, because I may fumble them.' This doesn't happen to a concert pianist, and it shouldn't happen to a surgeon. These are technical things that should be behind him by the time he gets to the operating room."

Dr. Kittle makes certain that he has taken all possibilities into account before he goes into surgery, reviewing technical points and discussing what is to be done with his associates. Along with cardiologists, radiologists and other specialists, he attends an hour-long briefing each Friday afternoon in which each operation scheduled for the next week is reviewed and questions of procedure are decided.

But plans don't always come to pass, and a surgeon must be ready for the unexpected. For this operation, Dr. Kittle had planned to use a valve from the hospital's frozen supply. But a "fresh" valve is preferable, and this morning at 7:30—with the patient already on the operating table—Dr. Kittle had received a telephone call at home telling him that a fresh valve was available.

A young Chicagoan had returned home the previous night to find his wife in bed with another man. In the ensuing fight, the husband received wounds from a butcher knife that proved fatal a few hours later.

The situation posed immediate problems. Getting permission from a coroner and a deceased person's next of kin takes time, as does removal of the organ for transplant. And the patient already was under anesthesia. "We don't like to keep patients asleep," Dr. Kittle explains. "It's an abnormal state and shouldn't be prolonged."

In this case, he says, "We couldn't locate the wife to get permission to use the valve because she had run away with the other guy. Ordinarily the nearest of kin has jurisdiction over the body and whenever possible we like to get the relative's permission. But if the nearest of relatives isn't available, and if it does involve homicide, then it becomes the jurisdiction of the coroner." The coroner gave permission, and Dr. Kittle decided to risk some delay and use the fresh valve.

He apparently relishes hard decisions. "The bigger the problem, the happier he is," says his wife, Jeane. Dr. El-Etr agrees. "One of his greatest features is that he doesn't panic under stress," says Dr. Kittle's associate. "Some surgeons swear, some shout or throw things. It doesn't take away from their skill, but it makes other people nervous. Dr. Kittle doesn't make other people nervous. I don't think anything in the operating room would make him lose control."

By 8:40 A.M., Dr. Kittle has begun to operate. He finishes opening the chest cavity and prepares to insert plastic tubes into the heart to link it to the heart-lung machine. At 9:05, Dr. Magdi H. Yacoub, another surgeon on the open-heart team, enters the operating room. He carries the homicide victim's heart, which he has just removed, in a stainless steel basin.

Now Dr. Yacoub begins the arduous task of cutting out the

valve from the dead man's heart and reinforcing it. Reinforcement is done with a piece of Dacron fastened around the outside of the valve. It takes nearly two hours, making Dr. Kittle slightly impatient. At 10:40, the job nearly done, the heart-lung machine is hooked up. It has a soft whirring and thumping rhythm.

Dr. Kittle makes the incision into the patient's heart. With a powerful vacuum device, Dr. Mizock swiftly sucks off gathering blood. Dr. Kittle cuts out the defective valve from the patient's heart, leaving a ragged-appearing hole for insertion of the new valve.

The next step requires painstaking patience. Using a needle holder that resembles a pair of long scissors, Dr. Kittle attaches the transplanted valve, carefully putting in more than 60 sutures. He labors for two hours within the confines of the four-inch incision.

"It's nice to watch his hands," says Dr. El-Etr. "He says he has always been clumsy, but in watching him operate, he doesn't look clumsy. He's very economical in his motions. He doesn't waste time with unnecessary maneuvers."

Dr. Kittle comments later: "The entire basis of surgery is what you can do with surgical techniques. So I think the most important thing for a surgeon is manual dexterity. People aren't going to be interested in surgery unless they like doing things with their hands."

Dr. Kittle does. As a child he studied the piano, and his parents gave him a grand piano during his school days that now stands in the living room of his Chicago apartment. Dr. Kittle still plays frequently, "usually late at night, mainly Beethoven sonatas," says Mrs. Kittle.

In the summers of his high school years, Dr. Kittle worked as a carpenter with his father, a contractor, building homes. "I think this building, working with one's hands, was such an integral part of my life," he says, "that it was only natural when I looked around for a profession to choose one where I could use my hands."

Now it is 12:30. The new valve is in place. "Okay, let's close this up and go home," Dr. Kittle says. In another 20 minutes the heart is closed. Then comes a delicate moment: Will the heart resume beating on its own when the heart-lung machine is turned off?

"We've all had the situation where every time we try to disconnect the heart-lung machine, the blood pressure gradually falls, the pulse speeds up and the heart isn't able to maintain a normal rhythm," Dr. Kittle says. "So then you go back on the pump and give whatever drugs you think are indicated. The heart may take over in a few hours, or it may not, and you have to call it quits." Turning off the pump for the final time is one of the heart surgeon's most painful decisions.

At 1:05 P.M., the ligatures on the great vessels feeding blood to the heart are loosened. The heart immediately begins to beat. Dr. Kittle eyes the wiggly yellow lines on the oscilloscope, which monitors heart beat and blood pressure. "His blood pressure looks great," the surgeon says. "He certainly came off the pump nicely."

But then another problem arises. As a plastic tube is withdrawn from the aorta, a jet of blood spurts out, striking an anesthesiologist in the face. The sutures are quickly pulled tight to close the hole. As the tension is released, there is a moment of levity while a nurse helps the anesthesiologist mop up. "That usually happens to me when I'm assisting," Dr. Kittle laughs.

The bleeding wasn't unexpected. But Dr. Robert L. Replogle, another heart surgeon, points out that a genuine error at this stage of surgery could be serious. "If you accidentally poke a hole in a blood vessel down in the abdomen," he says, "you've got no problem because you can sew it up quickly enough. But around the heart the vessels are much larger and blood pressure great, so if you poke a hole, it sprays the lights, the ceiling, everyone, and you've got real problems."

By 1:40 P.M., Dr. Kittle has closed the incision in the wall of the patient's chest. The senior resident takes over the final step, sewing up the skin. The operation has taken more than five hours. A heart transplant, by contrast, takes about two hours. It's not uncommon for Dr. Kittle to emerge from a long operation with a backache. "I probably don't have the table jacked up high enough," he jokes.

Often enough, there is emotional stress, too. Mrs. Kittle recalls the time about five years ago when her husband came home and wept after operating on the eight-year-old son of the milkman, a family friend. It was thought the boy had a congenital heart defect that could be corrected. The flaw turned out to be an unsuspected malformation that couldn't be repaired. The boy died on the operating table.

How does a surgeon feel at such a moment? "Someone once said it's not whether you win or lose, but how you play the game," Dr. Kittle comments. "In heart surgery, it's not how you play the game, but whether you win or lose. Intellectually, of course, I realize I can't win every time. But emotionally I want to. So when a patient dies I feel terribly dejected.

"Probably the first thought I have is, could I have done anything differently? Sometimes this is a black or white yes or no. Sometimes there are shades of gray. And in your development you quickly realize surgeons aren't infallible, that the medical profession isn't infallible.

"Then probably the second thought is, gee, how am I going to go down and explain this to the family? I think this bothers everybody. It's not an easy task. But, as Harry Truman said, 'if you don't like the heat, get out of the kitchen.' "

XIII

After the Attack

"Too often the forgotten person is the wife of the patient who has had a heart attack. She would not be much of a wife if she were not anxious and under stress. A study has just been made in London of 65 such wives because it was realized that the understanding, attitude and ability to cope may be crucial in the patient's rehabilitation."

So begins an item in an obscure little publication that circulates among people who have had attacks. It's called The Bulletin of the Coronary Club of Cleveland Inc. The "club" is a rather loose organization—it only meets once a year--of former heart attack victims who've run into a not uncommon frustration: trying to get their doctors to answer the myriad of seemingly trivial questions that plague a person's mind in the months following a heart attack. The Bulletin is the club's main raison d'etre.

At first glance the Bulletin looks like it might be an emploe publication put out by the personnel department of a rubber company, for by Madison Avenue standards it's rather amateurish.

By a check of the names of the editors and authors gives The Bulletin a different aura. The editor is Dr. Irvine H. Page who, until his retirement, was research director of the

famed Cleveland Clinic Foundation. The associate editors
are Dr. J. Willis Hurst, the Emory University heart
specialist who was physician to the late President Johnson,
and Dr. William L. Proudfit, head of cardiology at the
Cleveland Clinic. Past by-lines have included the late Dr.
Paul Dudley White, the Boston cardiologist who attended
President Eisenhower and Harvard nutritionist Dr. Frederick J. Stare.

Written in layman's language, The Bulletin is a kind of
combination Consumers Report, Dear Abby, and the Journal of the American Association, aimed at heart patients and
their families. The item about the problems of the wives of
heart patients, for example, illustrates how The Bulletin can
sum up the findings of a scientific study.

"The suddenness of the (husband's) illness caused a
sense of numbness, panic and feeling of unreality (among
the wives)," The Bulletin explains. " 'I feel I have lost the
strong husband I had.' Some wives felt guilty for things they
had or had not done. The feeling of loss, depression and
anxiety often produce sleep and appetite disturbances.
Some developed headaches, faintness and heart symptoms.

"After the husband left the hospital many wives found the
convalescent period very stressful due to 1) their sense of
loss and fear of recurrence and 2) problems associated with
the husband's return home. Wives were unsure whether
the recurrence of chest pain was serious or not. The husband often was dependent and irritable, resulting in tension
and over-hostility. If the wife expressed sympathy some
husbands became more helpless and demanding but if they
responded with firmness they (the wives) then felt guilty."

In its four printed pages readers will find personal accounts of heart attacks, hospitalization and recovery (Dr.
White once recounted how he experienced his first chest

pain at age 81 while rushing down Commonwealth Avenue in Boston to see the finish of the Boston Marathon); an evaluation of the cholesterol-lowering drug, Atromid-S (researchers are "too anxious" to report results for or against it so beware of newspaper stories about the drug); and suggestions about eating in resturants (concentrate heavily on salads "the only source of polyunsaturated oil is salad dressing and mayonnaise").

And there is some down-to-earth advice about interpreting newspaper stories relating to heart disease. Reports that heart attacks are less common, statistically, in areas that have "hard" water than localities with "soft" water can be misleading, The Bulletin cautions. "For instance, it was said at one time that the likelihood of having a heart attack was increased by having a television license in Great Britain," The Bulletin notes. Right now, it says, there's no reason for heart patients to throw away their softeners or worry about moving to hard water areas.

The Bulletin is the outgrowth of what Dr. Page describes as a rather embarrassing episode. In addition to his pioneering research on high blood pressure, Dr. Page for many years has been deep into the studies on the aspects of American life—diet, smoking, high blood pressure, overweight, inactivity, etc.—that seem to contribute to the nation's pandemic of heart attacks. Among other efforts, he was chairman of the National Cooperative Diet-Heart Study, a major experiment involving 1,500 middle-aged American men to see if Americans could switch over and stick to a low-fat, low-cholesterol diet.

The day after he chaired the final session of scientists who carried out the study and approved the final report, the cardiologist was stricken by a heart attack. No one was more surprised than Dr. Page, himself, since he steadfastly practiced his own preachments on a life style that would minimize the risks of a heart attack. It was a medium-sized attack involving only one of the coronary artery branches.

"I really can't describe what it felt like; I don't think anyone can," Dr. Page recalls. "It wasn't terribly painful and there wasn't any sense of impending death; it's a feeling in your chest you never had before and you know what it is when it happens," he says.

A few weeks later, a long time friend, U. A. Whitaker, then chairman of AMP Inc. of Harrisburg, Pa., dropped by to see Dr. Page. Since Mr. Whitaker himself had recovered from a heart attack several years previously, talk turned to what life was like after a heart attack.

"What struck him (Mr. Whitaker) was that I was in a far better situation than he had been" in understanding what had happened, Dr. Page recalls. Unlike the vast majority of heart attack patients who are mystified by their heart attacks, Dr. Page not only had his own extensive knowledge of the disease but anytime he had a question he could pick up the phone and talk to the nation's leading heart experts, all of whom are professional and personal friends.

Most people, including doctors, don't realize what goes through the mind of a person in the months following a heart attack, Dr. Page says. There's the problem of waking up in the middle of the night wondering when the second attack might occur, the fears of taking a business trip and staying alone in a hotel in a strange city, worries over what to eat and not to eat, concern over sexual relations and the quandaries over headlines about heart disease. "There's a lot of scare stuff that gets published (in the newspapers) and, when you're sensitized to it, it's rough," he explains.

Most heart patients hate to repeatedly pester their own doctors with such seemingly trivial questions or when they do their doctors often are too busy to give more than a

116

superficial "don't worry about it" answer. So why not get some of Dr. Page's medical friends to fill the gap?, Mr. Whitaker and Dr. Page decided.

Mr. Whitaker handled the organizational details of what became the Coronary Club and Dr. Page began talking his colleagues into writing a series of pamphlets. Several of the pamphlets are simply written pieces of advice on how to live with coronary artery disease usually with the doctor-authors telling how they treat their own heart patients.

The most popular pamphlets, however, are first-person accounts, often by physicians, of heart attacks. Dr. George C. Griffith, emeritus professor of medicine at the University of Southern California, once wrote a highly detailed description of his near-fatal heart attack and subsequent open-heart surgery, while Dr. Walter C. Bornemeier, past president of the American Medical Association, recalled how his attack struck while he was completing an operation.

The Bulletin follows the pattern of the pamphlets. It may include a personal account of a heart attack, another article by Dr. Proudfit describing a new type of surgery or discussing whether automobile driving is risky for the heart patient, a food column by Cleveland Clinic dietician Helen Brown, or a letter from someone like Speaker of the House, Rep. Carl Albert, who had a heart attack several years ago, agreeing to serve on the Club's honorary board (along with such notables as singer Pearl Bailey and actress Patricia Neal).

There are also some pithy comments, usually written by Dr. Page, that are reminiscent of the style of the country doctor. He once accused the airlines of adding to the dangers of their passengers having heart attacks:

"Look at the breakfast served by one of the best airlines," he wrote, "fruit (canned) cup, egg and cheese omelet, sweet roll dripping with butter and strong coffee. Add a cigaret before and after, complete immobility enforced by the seat belt, and you have a perfect plan to increase the cardiologist's business. . . . If the airlines were as careless in the feeding and maintenance of their planes as of their customers, their future would be dim indeed."

Another time, in mock despair over newspaper stories about causes and treatment of heart disease, The Bulletin declared "What next will be suggested? No one knows, perhaps mammoth doses of vitamin C, DDT, or 'soft' whiskey . . . Too bad medicine no longer resembles the days when half your ailments were cured by going to bed and the other half by getting up."

The Bulletin is put together strictly as a hobby by Dr. Page and his secretary, Ethel Strattan, and is published by the Coronary Club from its headquarters at 20310 Chagrin Boulevard (Cleveland 44122). There's no specific charge for it but recently its circulation reached the point where printing and postage bills were a bit high for the anonymous businessmen who had been supporting it. As a result, the Coronary Club has been asking but not requiring "dues" of anywhere from $3 to $50 a year, depending on a person's ability to pay.

XIV

A Patient's Chronicle

One strange facet of coronary disease is that medical scientists report their research findings by the reams in medical journals and physicians write about its prevention and treatment by the volumes. But seldom is the central object of this word torrent, the patient, heard from. Heart patients rarely talk about their experience, much less write about it.

In early 1974, however, the Coronary Club, Inc., in Cleveland, began distributing a fascinating account of one person's encounter with coronary disease and coronary surgery. It was written by Jane Rosenthal, 58-year-old writer and lecturer, and currently an editor of Bon Appetit magazine. She lives in Shawnee Mission, Kans.

Miss Rosenthal's chronicle:

"Women's Lib" has yet to make its well-justified way into the realm of coronary disease. The publicity given the Nation's No. 1 killer tends to portray it as a "for men only" ailment; nothing could be further from the truth. Somehow the nasty little statistic is overlooked that after fifty women are as vulnerable as men to coronary artery problems. Research is now proving that a surprising number of women are developing them at an even earlier age.

This is *my own* highly personal approach to the subject of

heart surgery and no two people react alike to a given set of circumstances. It is in the hope of helping others I have chosen to relive here the months of "trial by fire." In retrospect, however, I have much to be grateful for—the love and concern of family and friends, the devoted care of nurses and hospital attendants and above all the kindness and skill of an incomparable group of doctors. I am convinced it is by the grace of God and the work of these gifted people that I am alive today.

During such a long, drawn-out period, you have to learn to cope with change. Frequently there are career problems, but the world doesn't collapse around you. If you've raced through life and then must halt for an extended period, you find ambition has fled. Most trying of all is one's disposition. I'm often cross, grumpy and moody, but thank God for family and friends who unfailingly understand.

From two packs of cigarettes a day (sometimes more) to none; from gourmet cuisine to the bland, low-fat, low-cholesterol, low-calorie diet which now and ever shall make hunger a way of life; plus the imperative daily one to two mile walks—one's disposition does suffer. However, moments come when you are glad to be alive and enjoy the blue of the sky, the rolling waves of the ocean, the song of birds, a lovely passage from Mozart, a painting by Monet, the love of those close to you—these make the answer to the question, "is the anguish and pain of heart surgery worth it?" an unequivocal "YES."

Of course some days you will feel marvelous and others dreadful. You'll have bleak moments of depression, moments of fright when your heart pounds off-beat with such fury you wonder if each one may be the last. I still do, and it has been two years since my first angina attack and eighteen months since my three vein by-pass surgery. But knowing that others all around the world share the same feelings buoys the spirit tremendously.

Actually, very little has been written about open-heart surgery by patients . . . undoubtedly some prefer to block the episode from their minds . . . others, like myself, find it fascinating. Rachel McKenzie wrote a brief and moving book on her personal experience entitled, "Risk"; more recently James Cameron penned a gripping piece about his heart surgery in Harper's Magazine, called "Journal of a Trip to Limbo." As with travel books, which are best read after one returns (before, places unseen and unknown are unreal) most reading about heart surgery is best done some months later when the fright and pain have lessened considerably.

And make no mistake about it . . . heart surgery is terrifying. News items can give the heart patient distress and sleepless nights. This is just one of the highly commendable attributes of The Coronary Club Incorporated. Its wise, thoughtful physicians are there to answer the endless questions which tumble one after another through a patient's mind for months. During recovery, patients are reluctant to trouble their own over-worked doctors with each strange reaction and symptom.

The heart is a legendary symbol of love and sadness, happiness and despair. It can withstand an incredible amount of the punishment dealt it in the complex society of the mid-20th century. But it is rebelling more and more . . . there are too many massive coronaries that snuff out life in a brief moment, too many victims of myocardial infarction being rushed to the Intensive Care Unit . . . where happily a great many lives are saved.

Most of these patients return to their everyday lives, although altered by firm rules concerning diet, exercise and nicotine. Just a decade ago innumerable persons being saved by surgery today were giving up young, vital lives to a failing heart.

Surgery gives a reprieve. Above all you find yourself becoming enthusiastic about the operation itself, with a genuine interest in and support of the American Heart Association, The Coronary Club Incorporated, the Mended Hearts, Inc., and the relatively new, highly innovative Heart/Life, whose program is concentrated on the preventive aspect of coronary problems.

New surgical techniques and discoveries are being developed so fast . . . my tale of 1972 may already be outdated, but I suspect the basics will remain . . . the semi-artistic incision that meanders down the middle of your torso, a couple of inch long horizontal ones just below your ribs on the right and left sides, two moderately long ones on the inside of your thigh which allowed the removal of the very important vein required to repair your heart. You may still have a small white dot on your left wrist where the little funnel gave up varying amounts of blood to the technicians each day. The intravenous needle marks have disappeared but the arteriogram incision remains.

The weekly blood tests that continue after discharge while still on blood thinner leave an odd mark or two . . . you are something of a horror to yourself. But after eighteen months I find much of the cutting and stitching has faded and except for an occasional glance from a sales lady when buying a dress or blouse (the incision down the breast bone baffles them) I am in just about as good a condition as could be expected. The incision hurts and still disrupts my sleep at night . . . but two fine 24-hour FM radio stations help relieve the tedious business of lying awake.

The totally new diet and the deprivation of cigarettes are the most onerous remnants you must learn to live with, and I can recommend Greek worry beads and needlework when you think you cannot survive another minute without a cigarette. Nevertheless, this new life style for some may be a source of emotional upheaval.

Heart disease has many manifestations and often appears without warning. I'd just returned from a Christmas holiday in New England . . . my first non-working vacation in years. Typically, I'd had quantities of holiday fare (alcoholic and otherwise) smoked heavily as usual but spent some time out of doors and had never felt better . . . my job was happy and creatively satisfying. Secretly, I promised myself I'd lose weight, cut down on smoking and exercise each day, but the time was not yet.

I woke suddenly in the middle of the night a few weeks later with a terrific, grinding pain in my chest which radiated out to my shoulders, arms and hands as well as my throat and between my shoulder blades. I said to myself, "women don't have heart trouble," and dismissed it as indigestion. But the pain recurred night after night and lack of sleep was beginning to tell. Also the pains were beginning to come during the daytime so it seemed the better part of valor to see my internist. This good doctor had examined me regularly for 20 years and none of the former EKGs gave evidence of any major problem. The one he gave me that day showed no change, but the "Master-Two-Step" indicated clearly something was amiss. One snowy night a few days later I wound up in the emergency room at St. Luke's Hospital. A three-week stay consisted of tests, tests and more tests and finally a thorough (fine-tooth comb) examination by a leading cardiologist. I was already on a 900 calorie a day diet, had cut down on cigarettes and fully expected him to discharge me, but NO! Back to bed for at least two weeks with the stern admonition, "you are *never* to smoke another cigarette."

I Think I'm Having a Heart Attack

The doctors hoped the angina might be controlled medically, and I was discharged with a severe warning that too many repeat performances, extending over too long a time, meant an arteriogram to see what the difficulties really were. This is a rugged test but necessary to supply the answer if by-pass surgery is indicated and possible.

From January to May we tried medical treatment and since I was so scared it wasn't too difficult to drop close to 40 pounds and try to adjust to a dreadfully unpalatable diet, get some exercise and hardest of all . . . quit smoking entirely. The pain persisted, getting a little more severe each time. Nitroglycerin helped at first, but soon no longer relieved the pain. An arteriogram became necessary and once the results were in, I knew my time had come. The three major arteries in my heart were virtually closed and a coronary was at hand. My surgeon said if I chose to wait for a real heart attack, my chances of survival were fair, but the damage to the heart muscle would make the surgical procedure more difficult. If we could do the surgery before that damage was done, the percentages were infinitely more in my favor. The coronary by-pass operation is still in its infancy and no one can be sure if it prolongs life . . . what it does do however is to remove much of the pain of angina.

I'm frequently besieged by questions from those who are facing surgery because I've lived through it. Few (if any) of the surgeons have experienced it . . . brilliant, able and unbelievably skillful, they know what happens physiologically, but not how you feel.

I am sure your major questions are . . . what it is like? . . . will I feel better? . . . will I be able to return to my former life? . . . will life really be worth living? With a few minor qualifications, the answer is a resounding "Yes"!

The doctors and the head cardiological nurse give you

excellent preparatory information but if you are as terrified as I was, very little of it registers on your benumbed brain. They are enormously understanding and are on hand later when you can ask more intelligent questions.

I cannot stress too strongly that every individual is different and what touched and troubled me, you may well escape and vice versa . . . but this is *my* chronicle, and I sincerely hope some portion of it will be of help to you and your family.

In St. Luke's, Kansas City, where a skilled, brilliant and sympathetic man is head of cardiac surgery, open-heart operations proceed in a fairly classic manner with a fantastically low mortality rate. This surgeon and his team move like finely honed precision instruments.

As an "almost emergency" case, I had only two days (three or four are better) for the required preparations . . . massive doses of antibiotics, sessions with the head nurse, inhalation therapist, and anesthetist. The personnel manning the heart surgery floor are trained by surgeons and cardiologists. Like a skillful musical performance, the delicate surgery must be done over and over so that the doctors may keep the supple facility of movement in their hands. Much of the unfortunate publicity that seems to dog this promising operation is that too often it is performed irregularly. Where the hospital setting is at its best, the surgeon peerless, his team functioning to perfection, with an I.C.U. to back up both the surgeon and his patient, and with floor nurses and personnel equipped to handle recuperation, the heart patient has everything going for him. I can't and won't say that I'd go back for a repeat performance yet, but I suspect if it was necessary, I just might be able to make it!

Your hours in the operating room have a strange awareness and unreality. When you come to, you feel like a fractured marble statue. Aside from the pain, you've one sensation—COLD!

The Intensive Care Unit has to be classed as totally unbelievable. Even in the state of post-operative trauma the stay in I.C.U. (although you may owe your life to these alert medical shock troops) will probably be the most appalling experience you'll ever have. But even a modest knowledge of "what goes on in there" helps to a surprising degree.

From the strongest to the weakest character, I.C.U. takes preparation. It is a huge Hieronymous Bosch painting come to life. The tortures portrayed in works of this remarkable 15th century Dutch painter lead you to believe that Bosch foresaw what was in store for the heart surgery patient. On the plus side, I.C.U. is superb and patients are given constant, watchful care during those crucial 48 to 62 hours after operation (my supervisor caught fibrillation on my monitor and had the doctors there in a matter of minutes). Although it may seem forever, most patients spend a comparatively short time there. Still, were our Dutch friend to create a painting he'd have innumerable choices: the patient gasping and nearly suffocating in the clouds of cold oxygen pouring over his head, surrounded by bottles and tubes leading off into an unpenetrable fog; those irritating (but essential) little heart monitors that go "beep beep" while making odd abstract designs on a TV-like screen . . . that is, until you move the wrong way and the "beeps" become such a screech that the nurses come running. Bosch might well portray you as a solid block of ice because that is the way you feel; or, as expected and counted upon, enveloped in the flames of fever. Sleep comes only in fitful snatches . . . the lights burn constantly. If you do doze off the chances are you'll be awakened by a flashlight in your face amidst the vaporous clouds of oxygen. Off comes the tent and inhalation therapy begins . . . both are con-

126

tinued alternatively until you wonder if you are a victim of the Spanish Inquisition. Hope for any rest is short lived . . . you must sit up to cough, you must be weighed on a fantastic flat scale and endure that cold plate against your back for the daily chest X-ray.

Everyone's sojourn in I.C.U. produces a special set of memories . . . mine revolved around a raging thirst that was not to be slaked for so long it was easy to conjure up visions of the Sahara. One boon was that the icy oxygen condensed inside the tent and rolled down my face so that with luck I just might get a drop or two in my mouth. Thirst became a real obsession and I can still hear that never-ending leitmotif of pounds of ice cubes being poured into the oxygen machine. I can hear the clink of ice in glasses as attendants stopped by the ice maker. It was such an incredible experience that ICE will always be a special commodity to me.

Back in a regular hospital room, everything brightens . . . ghastly bottles and tubes are removed as is that annoying, ubiquitous monitor. The stitches come out (and that hurts) but you're getting food (bland and salt-free) and ice water finally. You feel less like a beetle pinned on a board. Then you are shakily on your feet.

One very tough experience is that day (carefully predicted in the advance briefing) when for no apparent reason you cry from morning to night. This and other emotional reactions are attracting research scholars. The heart is historically more than just an organ of the body . . . thus there must be some religious and metaphysical depths still to be explored.

The day arrives when you must face the fact that you are still alive. The pains in the chest, pounding flip-flops in the region of your heart cause you to wonder for how long. But, rest assured, your doctor would never dismiss you if you were not ready to start the long trek back to a useful life . . . not the one you lived before, but there are portents it can be an even better one.

An extremely effective key to the period of recuperation and rehabilitation is your cardiologist and his staff . . . mine I class as Saints all! Their patience, their kind and thoughtful management of seemingly endless problems meant very much indeed. This is a time, too, when psychological problems may arise . . . during sleepless nights you linger on all that has happened; written words about heart surgery (good and bad) set off an alarm system that rakes your nerves . . . you feel sorry for yourself and deplore your new life style. I "psyched out" about two months after surgery. Postoperative depression, while fairly common, does not always develop. My personal bout with depression, inability to concentrate and general malaise hasn't been easy to solve, but a top psychiatrist can help restore your mental health and lead you back to a measure of self-confidence and self-reliance, two attributes which have deserted you entirely. Working with a psychiatrist, the hospital chaplains and/or the rector of your church, you have a powerful team . . . call on them for help. You'll never regret it.

Well on the road to recovery, it is the grateful heart patient to whom this saying, attributed to Etienne de Grellet, means the most, because you've found you've become a real crusader. . . . "I expect to pass through this world but once; any good thing therefore that I can do; or any kindness that I can show any fellow creature, let me do it now, let me not defer or neglect it, for I shall not pass this way again." Making this motto an important part of your life and living up to it, you'll know you've come through a remarkable surgical experience with all flags flying.

XV

In the Future, a New Heart

When the headlines mushroomed up from Cape Town, South Africa, in late 1967, proclaiming the world's first human heart transplant, the world was agog. Not only did the feat involve the organ long viewed as the center of life, it heralded the new era of cure for Western society's biggest killer. In a matter of months surgical teams around the globe and particularly in the United States were transplanting hearts almost on a weekly basis, whenever chance brought together in the same medical center a newly dead donor and a dying recipient.

Today the transplantation of the human heart seems to lie in limbo. No longer are these dramatic operations being done in Texas, Minnesota, Virginia, New York or other places that once were the datelines of front-page newspaper stories. The transplantation of kidneys, occasionally of the liver or the lungs sporadically break into the news, but not the heart.

There is an exception and a significant one. At Stanford University Medical Center in Palo Alto, Calif., a human heart is being transplanted on the average of once a month. It is being done without the glare of klieg lights or the clamor of headlines. There is neither controversy about the ethics of the heart transplants nor extravagant claims of success.

But if one were to follow closely the reports of the Stanford specialists that periodically are made to scientific gatherings or published in medical journals it would become clear that the heart transplant, far from being abandoned, is moving steadily closer to becoming an accepted treatment that eventually may save thousands of lives. With each successive report the number of persons alive with transplanted hearts grows.

This situation of Stanford continuing to do heart transplants while others seemingly have abandoned the operation isn't due to medical or scientific decisions. Rather, say the surgeons, it's a matter of public attitude.

In most areas in 1968 and 1969, whenever a heart transplant was performed at a medical center, the local press headlined the event and then followed the patient's progress almost day by day. More often than not, the patient died. in a matter of weeks, or a few months, an event that also was headlined.

As a result of this repeated reporting of deaths of transplant patients a widespread public disillusionment set in. Dr. Denton Cooley, the famed Houston heart surgeon who performed several heart transplants, appraising the situation in late 1972, noted that potential recipients "are saying to themselves, 'What's the use of a transplant? It only means a few months of life anyway.' This attitude rubs off on families of potential donors of hearts."

Thus, even in the increasingly rare instances of a dying person's being willing to receive a new heart, there aren't any hearts being offered.

In the Palo Alto-San Francisco area, however, the situation is considerably different. "When we did our first transplant (early 1968) there was a newspaper strike," recalls Dr.

Norman E. Shumway, head of the surgical team that performs the transplants and generally credited with having developed the surgical technique used for heart transplants. Since then the local press, notably the San Francisco Chronicle, the area's largest newspaper, has refused to sensationalize the transplants.

"We made an early decision not to go overboard," explains David Perlman, the Chronicle's science correspondent. The personal lives and the deaths of the patients weren't played up in the newspaper. "We focused on the donors only when the purpose was to increase the donation of organs," Mr. Perlman says. The Chronicle's coverage of heart transplants is devoted largely to the scientific results of the Stanford research.

Thus, the Stanford group continues to receive both willing recipients of hearts and donations of hearts. (For much the same reason, the San Francisco Bay area is a leader in the donation of kidneys for transplantation.)

By early 1974, Dr. Donald C. Harrison of the Stanford team was able to report "we have performed 65 cardiac transplants since January, 1968. We continue at the rate of approximately one transplant per month, and at the present time have 22 surviving patients."

More important, though, the length of time the transplant patients are living after their surgery is increasing steadily. Among the patients transplanted in that first year, 1968, only 22% survived for a year. For those transplanted in 1971, the one-year survival rate was up to 50%.

Using statistical methods of life-insurance actuaries, the Stanford specialists now calculate that if a transplant patient can survive the first critical three months, then his chances of living one year stand at 78%, of living two years at 68% and three years at 40%. Considering the fact that if a victim hadn't undergone the transplant, his chances of dying within six months were almost 100%, the Stanford figures are rather remarkable.

One reason for the improved survival rates is that the Stanford researchers are learning to more carefully select patients who are likely to benefit from the transplant. Firstly, of course, they pick only people who otherwise are likely to soon die from a severely damaged or failing heart. About 70% of the transplant recipients are endangered by coronary artery disease while the rest suffer other heart ailments.

Initially, some health authorities put the number of "good" candidates for heart transplants in the U.S. at 80,000 to 90,000 a year, an estimate that would have required an appalling number of heart donations. The Stanford experience, however, has indicated that this is a vast overestimate. Several groups of heart patients just aren't good candidates for transplants.

The elderly seem to be among these high-risk groups, partly because they have difficulty withstanding the onslaught of infections that threaten a transplant patient because of the immunity-suppressing drugs used to prevent rejection of his new heart. Therefore, the Stanford surgeons tend to restrict transplants to patients in the mid-50's or younger.

Similarly, a person who has had severe, crippling heart disease for longer than five years isn't a good candidate. This is particularly true if the heart disease has caused the blood vessels in the lungs to become callused and narrowed. Such a condition forces the lower right chamber of the heart to work increasingly harder to force blood through these narrowed vessels in the lungs. This pressure load on the lower right chamber can become so great that even the healthy transplanted heart can't bear up and the transplant fails, sometimes in a matter of hours after surgery.

In the Future, a New Heart

"A heart transplant isn't for everybody," says Dr. Shumway.

However, only part of the center's increasing survival rate can be laid to more careful selection of transplant recipients. Another reason is the discovery—and, it's hoped, the conquest—of a problem that seems to strike the new heart once transplanted.

It seems that the underlying coronary artery disease that led to the need for a heart transplant in the first place, or something much like the disease, may afflict the transplanted heart and do so extremely rapidly. Before they transplant a heart, the surgeons try to make sure the new organ is free of the clogging deposits of coronary artery disease.

"In the first six long-term (a year or more) survivors of cardiac transplantation who later expired, a major form of coronary atherosclerosis was detected in the new heart," says Dr. Harrison. "This atherosclerosis appeared to be an accelerated form of the standard variety of coronary artery disease we observe in thousands of patients each year." Deposits in the coronaries that normally take years to build up were piling up in the transplanted hearts in months.

Just why this happens so rapidly in a transplanted heart isn't known. One theory of the Stanford scientists as well as other researchers, explains Dr. Harrison, is that the body's attempt to reject the foreign heart somehow damages the inner walls of the coronary arteries. It is this damage that leads to a rapid build-up of fatty deposits on the artery walls. (The researchers are trying to find out if a similar process lies behind the coronary artery disease that afflicts the "native" heart; if so, the discovery would be a major scientific "fall-out" of heart transplantation research.)

Whatever the cause, the Stanford researchers, beginning in early 1970 with their 17th transplant, have been pressing their patients to strictly follow a regimen that most doctors prescribe for their heart-attack patients. They are told to lose their excess weight, and their diet is sharply restricted in saturated fats and cholesterol.

In addition, anticoagulants, drugs that help to prevent blood clots, are taken regularly. The patient checks in every two months for an electrocardiogram, and he comes in annually for a special X-ray—coronary arteriography—that can determine whether coronary arteries are beginning to clog up.

The effort appears to be paying off. Of the patients who have been on the treatment long enough for it to make a difference, almost all are free of coronary artery deposits. Moreover, the Stanford surgeons believe, if the coronaries do start clogging up, the bi-monthly X-ray will spot it before it reaches the stage of heart failure or a heart attack. The patient then might be a candidate for a second heart transplant.

The Stanford team, with its growing experience, also has learned how to spot, at an early stage, when the body is attempting to reject the new heart. Often, particularly after the first three months, this rejection phenomenon will seem to be dormant or, at least, under control. Then, suddenly it will spring to life. The rejection, of course, would be fatal unless doctors can suppress it in time with drugs.

The Stanford group has learned there are a number of abnormalities that occur when the rejection process is in its earliest phases. The wall of the heart, for instance, begins to swell and stiffen, and, as the body begins trying to destroy the "foreign" heart tissue, the heart develops mechanical abnormalities. The mechanical changes can be spotted early with some new techniques such as echocardiography, a sonar-like method of bouncing sound waves off the heart.

Improving on a technique initially developed in Japan,

the Stanford scientists also can take tiny samples of the transplanted heart. A tiny set of pincers is mounted on the tip of a catheter. By making a small opening in a vein in the neck, the pincer-tipped catheter can be advanced into the heart where a tiny piece of heart tissue is nipped off, painlessly, and removed. The tissue can then be studied under the electron microscope and in the chemistry laboratory for changes that signal the beginning of a rejection episode.

"This has proven to be a safe method to biopsy the inner surface of the heart and is now routinely used in all cardiac transplant patients," Dr. Harrison says. (Some of these same techniques are being turned toward the study of heart disease generally, another "fall-out" benefit of heart transplantation, Dr. Harrison says.)

Doctors can control these rejection episodes, especially when they are spotted in their incipient stages. But, to do so, they must tread a thin line. The immunity-suppressing drugs are capable of knocking out the body's immune system totally. While this is done in the first weeks after surgery while in the hospital, it can't be done month after month or the patient would be totally defenseless against infections. Thus, the drugs have to be given in dosages that will prevent the immune system from attacking the new heart but still leave some immune defenses against germs and viruses.

The real breakthrough that would open up the use of heart transplantation to its fullest, scientists say, would be some way of selectively disabling the immune system. "We're still looking for the magic drug, one that will keep the body from rejecting the new heart but leave the rest of the immune system intact," explains one transplant expert.

What is it like to have a transplanted heart?

James Marshall, a short, ebullient interior decorator from Mountain View, Calif., talked briefly about this in the fall of

135

1972. Three years earlier, at age 48, Mr. Marshall had, without warning, suffered a heart attack so damaging that it seemed he had little chance of living more than a few months. He went on the Stanford center's waiting list and, after several weeks, received the fateful telephone call that the heart of a 22-year-old woman was available for transplantation.

Shortly before the third anniversary of receiving the new heart, Mr. Marshall was able to complain that his biggest problem "is my diet; I'm five pounds overweight." He was not only back to working full time but was making speeches about his transplant to civic groups and the like at the rate of two to five a month.

"My friends sometimes treat me as though I were fragile, that my heart was going to break," he noted. Otherwise, his life, if anything, is more active than before, he says.

Nevertheless, Lois K. Christopherson, chief social worker for the Stanford surgery department, who has studied and tried to help transplant recipients, reports they do have psychological problems. "Even after the patient is discharged to return to an amazingly normal, active life style," she says, "he is reminded of his tenuous hold on life by the publicly reported deaths of other transplant survivors."

XVI

The Turning Point

In 1971 the U.S. Government Printing Office issued a large, blue hard-cover book priced at $6.95. Like most of the GPO publications it is hardly entertaining reading. But in a subtly significant way the volume signals a turning point in man's conquest of disease.

The book is titled simply Cardiovascular Diseases, Guidelines for Prevention and Care. It signifies that perhaps for the first time in history enough is known about a chronic disease for people to begin thinking realistically of its elimination.

"It is essential that plans now be formulated for a concerted attack on these (cardiovascular) diseases during the 1970's, if we are to reduce the tragic death and disability they cause throughout the nation," the introduction declares. "Improvement in this situation will result in major social and economic gains from the productivity and leadership of the many who otherwise will be stricken before or during their most productive years."

The book is the product of the Inter-Society Commission on Heart Disease Resources, organized by the American Heart Association and financed by a Federal grant. Under the chairmanship of New York heart and stroke specialist

Dr. Irving S. Wright and project director Dr. Donald T. Fredrickson, more than 150 heart disease experts from 29 medical organizations spent months pulling together the available knowledge on coronary and other heart diseases and then mapping a plan on what resources are needed to put the knowledge to use.

This in sharp contrast to the struggle against other chronic diseases. The well-funded "Conquest of Cancer" program now under way is still concentrated in the laboratory; with the exception of the now-proven link between lung cancer and smoking, the prevention and treatment of cancer remains basically unchanged from the 1940's. Arthritis, to name another chronic disease, continues to be a frustrating mystery as is multiple sclerosis, muscular dystrophy and mental retardation.

But to the Inter-Society Commission the means are now at hand to drastically reduce deaths from heart diseases, particularly coronary artery disease. To cite a few of its recommendations:

"The commission recommends that a strategy of primary prevention of premature atherosclerotic diseases be adopted as a long-term national policy for the United States and to implement this strategy that adequate resources of money and manpower be committed to accomplish:

. . . Changes in diet to prevent or control hyperlipidemia (high blood fat), obesity, hypertension and diabetes,

. . . Elimination of cigaret smoking,

. . . Pharmacologic (drug) control of elevated blood pressure."

Total elimination of these three risk factors would prevent 300,000 heart attacks and 60,000 deaths annually, the commission calculates.

As to the heart attack victim, himself, the commission

138

declares: "Because preventable deaths are occurring before patients reach medical attention, the delay between onset of symptoms and the establishment of effective monitoring and therapy must be shortened."

Thus, it urges the use of the specially equipped coronary care ambulances and helicopters along with special "life support units" in emergency rooms that can keep the patient alive until he can be rushed into the coronary care ward. The coronary care wards, themselves, are of "undisputed value" but, it cautions against every hospital in a community trying to establish these expensive coronary care units. A coronary care unit that isn't staffed and used 24 hours a day may dwindle into less-than-optimum care and "give a hospital and a community a false sense of security and may actually increase the risk to the patient."

Instead, communities and hospitals ought to get together and set up only one or two first-class coronary care units to which all hospitals in the area will refer patients. In addition, new "regional reference centers" should be set up. These would be able to carry out the newest and most elaborate of procedures ranging from the installation of pacemakers to coronary arteriography to implanting artificial heart pumps.

The value of surgery for coronary artery disease is still uncertain and no one can predict how many patients will need it and how many new open-heart surgical units will have to be set up, the commission says. To avoid low-quality care and surgery by inexperienced surgeons, however, the commission urges that such operations be done only in hospitals and medical centers that do a minimum of six open-heart operations a week.

There remains a host of unanswered questions about coronary disease, the commission says. It's not known, for example, precisely why and how fats in the diet, cholesterol in the blood and clogging of the arteries are related. Nor, for that matter, why and how smoking, diabetes, psychological tensions increase the risk of heart attacks.

"The question of genetic traits has been sadly neglected," the commission says. It's well known that heart attacks are extremely common in certain families but no one knows why. Nor is there much known about the role of hormones in protecting women in their premenopausal years against heart attacks.

The use of drugs in treating coronary disease is still a largely unexplored area. "If the development of atherosclerosis can be significantly retarded or prevented the impact will be of major order," the report notes.

And so the commission continues through several pages citing question after question about coronary disease. Clearly the battle is far from over.

The preceding chapters in this book might seem to imply that the conquest of the heart attack is taking place in the laboratory and the hospital. But the war really will be won on a different front, as Dr. Wright notes in his introduction to the Inter-Society Commission report:

"It has become increasingly clear that the first line of defense of medical care is the informed patient and his family. If the individual does not understand what he must do to preserve health, and if he does not recognize when there is need of help, and if he is not prepared to take the appropriate steps to obtain this help, all of the world's medical knowledge will be of little value."

GLOSSARY

Heart Terms

These definitions are from A HANDBOOK OF HEART TERMS prepared by the U.S. Department of Health, Education and Welfare:

ADRENALIN

One of the secretions of two small glands, called adrenal glands, located just above the kidneys. This secretion, also called epinephrine, and sometimes prepared synthetically, constricts the small blood vessels (arterioles), increases the rate of heart beat, and raises blood pressure. It is called a vasoconstrictor or vasopressor substance.

AGE-ADJUSTED DEATH RATE

Also called age-adjusted mortality rate. Death rates which have been standardized for age for the purpose of making comparisons between different populations or within the same population at various intervals of time.

141

AGE-SPECIFIC DEATH RATE

Also called age-specific mortality rate. The ratio of deaths in a specific age group to the population of the same age group during a given period of time, such as a year. It is calculated by dividing the deaths that occurred among the specific age group during the year, by the mid-year population in the same group (estimated population in the age group on July 1) of the same year.

AMINE

An organic compound that may be derived from ammonia by the replacement of one or more of the hydrogen atoms by hydrocarbon radicals.

ANEURYSM

A spindle-shaped or sac-like bulging of the wall of a vein or artery, due to weakening of the wall by disease or an abnormality present at birth.

ANGINA PECTORIS

Literally means chest pain. A condition in which the heart muscle receives an insufficient blood supply, causing pain in the chest, and often in the left arm and shoulder. Commonly results when the arteries supplying the heart muscle (coronaries) are narrowed by atherosclerosis. *See Coronary Atherosclerosis.*

ANGIOCARDIOGRAPHY

X-ray examination of the heart and great blood vessels that follows the course of an opaque fluid which has been injected into the blood stream.

ANOREXIA

Lack or loss of appetite for food.

ANOXIA

Literally, no oxygen. This condition most frequently occurs when the blood supply to a part of the body is completely cut off. This results in the death of the affected tissue. For example, a specific area of the heart muscle may die when the blood supply (and hence the oxygen supply) has been blocked, as by a clot in the artery supplying that area.

ANTICOAGULANT

A drug which delays clotting of the blood. When given in cases of a blood vessel plugged up by a clot, it tends to prevent new clots from forming, or the existing clots from enlarging, but does not dissolve an existing clot. Examples are heparin and coumarin derivatives.

ANTIHYPERTENSIVE AGENTS

Drugs which are used to lower blood pressure such as rauwolfia, reserpine, veratrum, hydralazine, hexamethonium chloride, and many others.

ANXIETY

A feeling of apprehension, the source of which is unrecognized.

AORTA

The main trunk artery which receives blood from the lower left chamber of the heart. It originates from the base of the heart, arches up over the heart like a cane handle, and passes down through the chest and abdomen in front of the spine. It gives off many lesser arteries which conduct blood to all parts of the body except the lungs.

AORTIC ARCH

The part of the aorta or large artery leaving the heart, which curves up like the handle of a cane over the top of the heart.

AORTIC INSUFFICIENCY

An improper closing of the valve between the aorta and the lower left chamber of the heart admitting a back flow of blood.

AORTIC STENOSIS

A narrowing of the valve opening between the lower left chamber of the heart and the large artery called the aorta. The narrowing may occur at the valve itself or slightly above or below the valve. Aortic stenosis may be the result of scar tissue forming after a rheumatic fever infection, or may have other causes.

AORTIC VALVE

Valve at the junction of the aorta, or large artery, and the lower left chamber of the heart. Formed by three cup-shaped membranes called semilunar valves, it allows the blood to flow from the heart into the artery and prevents a back flow.

AORTOGRAPHY

X-ray examination of the aorta (main artery conducting blood from the lower left chamber of the heart to the body) and its main branches. This is made possible by the injection of a dye which is opaque to X-rays.

APEX

The blunt rounded end of the heart, directed downward, forward, and to the left.

APOPLEXY

Frequently called apoplectic stroke or simply a stroke. A sudden interruption of the blood supply to a part of the brain caused by the obstruction or rupture of an artery. Initially may be manifested by a loss of consciousness, sensation, or voluntary motion, and may leave a part of the body (frequently one side) temporarily or permanently paralyzed.

ARRHYTHMIA

An abnormal rhythm of the heart beat.

ARTERIAL BLOOD

Oxygenated blood. The blood is oxygenated in the lungs, passes from the lungs to the left side of the

145

heart via the pulmonary veins. It is then pumped by the left side of the heart into the arteries which carry it to all parts of the body. *See Venous Blood.*

ARTERIOLES

The smallest arterial vessels (about 0.2 mm. or $1/125$ inch in diameter) resulting from repeated branching of the arteries. They conduct the blood from the arteries to the capillaries.

ARTERIOSCLEROSIS

Commonly called hardening of the arteries. This is a generic term which includes a variety of conditions which cause the artery walls to become thick and hard and lose elasticity. *See Atherosclerosis.*

ARTERY

Blood vessels which carry blood away from the heart to the various parts of the body. They usually carry oxygenated blood except for the pulmonary artery which carries unoxygenated blood from the heart to the lungs for oxygenation. *See Vein.*

ASCHOFF BODIES

Spindle-shaped nodules, occurring most frequently in the tissue of the heart, often formed during an attack of rheumatic fever. Named after Ludwig Aschoff (1866–1942), a German pathologist who described them.

ATHEROMA

A deposit of fatty (and other) substances in the inner lining of the artery wall, characteristic of atherosclerosis. Plural form of the word is atheromata (ather-o-mah'ta). *See Atherosclerosis.*

ATHEROSCLEROSIS

A kind of arteriosclerosis in which the inner layer of the artery wall is made thick and irregular by deposits of a fatty substance. These deposits (called atheromata) project above the surface of the inner layer of the artery, and thus decrease the diameter of the internal channel of the vessel. *See Arteriosclerosis.*

ATRIAL SEPTUM

Sometimes called inter-atrial septum or inter-auricular septum. Muscular wall dividing left and right upper chambers of the heart which are called atria. *See Septum.*

ATRIO-VENTRICULAR BUNDLE

Also called Bundle of His, auriculo-ventricular bundle, or A-V bundle. A bundle of specialized muscle fibers running from a small mass of muscular fibers (atrioventricular node) between the upper chambers of the heart, down to the lower chambers. It is the only known direct muscular connection between the upper and lower heart chambers, and serves to conduct impulses for the rhythmic heart beat from the atrioventricular node to the heart muscle.

147

ATRIO-VENTRICULAR NODE

A small mass of special muscular fibers at the base of the wall between the two upper chambers of the heart. It forms the beginning of the Bundle of His which is the only known direct muscular connection between the upper and the lower chambers of the heart. The electrical impulses controlling the rhythm of the heart are generated by the pacemaker, conducted through the muscle fibers of the right upper chamber of the heart to the atrio-ventricular node, and then conducted to the lower chambers of the heart by the Bundle of His. *See Bundle of His.*

ATRIO-VENTRICULAR VALVES

The two valves, one in each side of the heart, between the upper and lower chamber. The one in the right side of the heart is called the tricuspid valve, and the one in the left side is called the mitral valve.

ATRIUM

One of the two upper chambers of the heart. Also called auricle, although this is now generally used to describe only the very tip of the atrium. Right atrium receives un-oxygenated blood from body. Left atrium receives oxygenated blood from lungs. Capacity in adult about 57 cc.

AUENBRUGGER, LEOPOLD JOSEPH (1722–1809)

Austrian physician who invented the technique of tapping the surface of the body to determine the condition of organs beneath. The technique is called percussion.

AURICLE

The upper chamber in each side of the heart. "Atrium" is another term commonly used for this chamber.

AURICULAR SEPTUM

Sometimes called inter-auricular septum or, more properly, inter-atrial septum. Muscular wall dividing left and right upper chambers of the heart which are called atria. *See Septum.*

AURICULO-VENTRICULAR BUNDLE

See Bundle of His.

AUSCULTATION

The act of listening to sounds within the body, usually with a stethoscope.

AUTONOMIC NERVOUS SYSTEM

Sometimes called involuntary nervous system or vegetative nervous system, it controls tissues not under voluntary control, e.g., glands, heart, and smooth muscles.

A-V BUNDLE

See Bundle of His.

149

BACTERIAL ENDOCARDITIS

An inflammation of the inner layer of the heart caused by bacteria. The lining of the heart valves is most frequently affected. It is most commonly a complication of an infectious disease, operation, or injury.

BALLISTOCARDIOGRAM

A tracing of the movements of the body caused by the beating of the heart. The instrument which records these movements is called a ballistocardiograph.

BALLISTOCARDIOGRAPH

An apparatus for recording the movements of the body caused by the beating of the heart.

BARBITURATE

A class of drugs which produce a calming effect. A sedative.

BENZOTHIADIAZINE

A drug used to increase the output of urine by the kidney. A diuretic.

BICUSPID VALVE

Usually called mitral valve. A valve of two cusps or triangular segments, located between the upper and lower chambers in the left side of the heart.

BLOOD PRESSURE

The pressure of the blood in the arteries.

1. Systolic blood pressure. Blood pressure when the heart muscle is contracted (systole).

2. Diastolic blood pressure. Blood pressure when the heart muscle is relaxed between beats (diastole). Blood pressure is generally expressed by two numbers, as 120/80, the first representing the systolic, and the second, the diastolic pressure.

BLUE BABIES

Babies having a blueness of skin (cyanosis) caused by insufficient oxygen in the arterial blood. This often indicates a heart defect, but may have other causes such as premature birth or impaired respiration.

BRADYCARDIA

Abnormally slow heart rate. Generally, anything below 60 beats per minute is considered bradycardia.

BRIGHT, RICHARD (1789–1858)

English physician who demonstrated the association of heart disease with kidney disease.

BROMIDE

Any one of several drugs which produce a calming effect. A sedative.

BUNDLE OF HIS

Also called auriculo-ventricular bundle, atrio-ventricular bundle, or A-V bundle. A bundle of specialized muscle fibers running from a small mass of muscular fibers (atrio-ventricular node) between the upper chambers of the heart, down to the lower chambers. It is the only known direct muscular connection between the upper and lower heart chambers, and serves to conduct impulses for the rhythmic heart beat from the atrio-ventricular node to the heart muscle. Named after Wilhelm His, German anatomist.

CAESALPINUS, ANDREAS (1519?–1603)

First to use the term "circulation" in connection with the movement of the blood. However, he still believed in many of the classical theories taught by Galen.

CALORIE

Sometimes called large or kilo-calorie. Unit used to express food energy. The amount of heat required to raise the temperature of 1 kilogram of water 1 degree Centigrade.

A high caloric diet has a prescribed caloric value above the total daily energy requirement. A low caloric diet has a prescribed caloric value below the total energy requirement.

CAPILLARIES

Extremely narrow tubes forming a network between the arterioles and the veins. The walls are composed of a single layer of cells through which oxygen and nutritive materials pass out to the tissues, and carbon dioxide and waste products are admitted from the tissues into the blood stream.

CARDIAC

Pertaining to the heart. Sometimes refers to a person who has heart disease.

CARDIAC CYCLE

One total heart beat, i.e., one complete contraction and relaxation of the heart. In man, this normally occupies about 0.85 second.

CARDIAC OUTPUT

The amount of blood pumped by the heart per minute.

CARDIOVASCULAR

Pertaining to the heart and blood vessels.

CARDIOVASCULAR-RENAL DISEASE

Disease involving the heart, blood vessels, and kidneys.

CARDITIS

Inflammation of the heart.

153

CAROTID ARTERIES

The left and right common carotid arteries are the principal arteries supplying the head and neck. Each has two main branches, external carotid artery and internal carotid artery.

CAROTID BODY

A small oval mass of cells and nerve endings about 5 mm. or $1/5$ inch long located in the carotid sinus —that is, at the branching point in the arteries supplying blood to the head and neck. The cells respond to chemical changes in the blood by causing changes in the rate of breathing, and certain other body changes. When the oxygen content of the blood is reduced, the carotid body causes an increase in respiration rate.

CAROTID SINUS

A slight dilation at the point where the internal carotid artery branches from the common carotid artery. The carotid arteries are those arteries which supply blood to the head and neck. The carotid sinus contains special nerve end organs which respond to a change in blood pressure by causing a change in the rate of heart beat. External pressure on the carotid sinus by stimulating some of the nerves in the sinus can also cause a drop in blood pressure and faintness.

CATHETER

A cardiac catheter is a diagnostic device for taking samples of blood, or pressure readings within the heart chambers which might reveal defects in the heart. It is a thin tube of woven plastic or other material to which blood will not adhere, which is inserted in a vein or artery, usually in the arm, and threaded into the heart. The catheter is guided by the physician who watches its progress by means of X-rays falling on a fluorescent screen. Catheters are also used to enter other tubular organs.

CATHETERIZATION
In cardiology, the process of examining the heart by means of introducing a thin tube (catheter) into a vein or artery and passing it into the heart.

CEREBRAL VASCULAR ACCIDENT
Sometimes called cerebrovascular accident, apoplectic stroke, or simply stroke. An impeded blood supply to some part of the brain, generally caused by one of the following four conditions:

1. a blood clot forming in the vessel (cerebral thrombosis)

2. a rupture of the blood vessel wall (cerebral hemorrhage)

3. a piece of clot or other material from another part of the vascular system which flows to the brain and obstructs a cerebral vessel (cerebral embolism)

4. pressure on a blood vessel as by a tumor.

CEREBROVASCULAR
Pertaining to the blood vessels in the brain.

CHAGAS HEART DISEASE
A form of heart disease resulting from an infection by a microscopic parasite found in South America.

CHEMOTHERAPY
The treatment of disease by administering chemicals. Frequently used in the phrase "chemotherapy of hypertension," i.e., the treatment of high blood pressure by the use of drugs.

CHLORAL HYDRATE
A drug, which has a calming action, used to induce sleep. A sedative.

CHLOROTHIAZIDE
A chemical compound which increases the output of urine. One of the diuretics sometimes used in the treatment of edema, or water-logged tissues.

CHOLESTEROL
A fat-like substance found in animal tissue. In blood tests the normal level for Americans is assumed to be between 180 and 230 milligrams per 100 cc. A higher level is often associated with high risk of coronary atherosclerosis.

CHORDAE TENDINEAE
Fibrous chords which serve as guy ropes to hold the valves between the upper and lower chambers of the

heart secure when forced closed by pressure of blood in the lower chambers. They stretch from the cusps of the valves to muscles called papillary muscles in the walls of the lower heart chambers.

CHOREA

Involuntary, irregular twitching of the muscles sometimes associated with rheumatic fever. Also called St. Vitus Dance, or Sydenham's Chorea.

CIRCULATORY

Pertaining to the heart, blood vessels, and the circulation of the blood.

CLAUDICATION

Pain and lameness or limping caused by defective circulation of the blood in the vessels of the limbs.

CLUBBED FINGERS

Fingers with a short broad tip and overhanging nail, somewhat resembling a drumstick. This condition is sometimes seen in children born with certain kinds of heart defects.

COAGULATION

Process of changing from a liquid to a thickened or solid state. The formation of a clot.

COARCTATION OF THE AORTA

Literally a pressing together, or a narrowing of the aorta which is the main trunk artery which conducts blood from the heart to the body. One of several types of congenital heart defects.

COLLATERAL CIRCULATION

Circulation of the blood through nearby smaller vessels when a main vessel has been blocked up.

COMMISSUROTOMY

An operation to widen the opening in a heart valve which has become narrowed by scar tissue. The individual flaps of the valve are cut or spread apart along the natural line of their closure. This operation often performed in cases of rheumatic heart disease. *See Mitral Valvulotomy.*

COMPENSATION

A change in the circulatory system made to compensate for some abnormality. An adjustment of size of heart or rate of heart beat made to counterbalance a defect in structure or function. Often used specifically to describe the maintenance of adequate circulation in spite of the presence of heart disease.

CONGENITAL ANOMALY

An abnormality present at birth.

CONGESTIVE HEART FAILURE

When the heart is unable adequately to pump out all the blood that returns to it, there is a backing up of blood in the veins leading to the heart. A congestion or accumulation of fluid in various parts of the body (lungs, legs, abdomen, etc.) may result from the heart's failure to maintain a satisfactory circulation. *See Myocardial Insufficiency.*

CONSTRICTION

Narrowing, as in the phrase "vaso-constriction," which is a narrowing of the internal diameter of the blood vessels, caused by a contraction of the muscular coat of the vessels.

CONSTRICTIVE PERICARDITIS

A shrinking and thickening of the outer sac of the heart which prevents the heart muscle from expanding and contracting normally.

CONTRACTILE PROTEINS

The protein substance within the heart muscle fibers responsible for heart contraction by shortening the muscle fibers.

CORONARY ARTERIES

Two arteries, arising from the aorta, arching down over the top of the heart, and conducting blood to the heart muscle.

CORONARY ATHEROSCLEROSIS

Commonly called coronary heart disease. An irregular thickening of the inner layer of the walls of the arteries which conduct blood to the heart muscle. The internal channel of these arteries (the coronaries) becomes narrowed and the blood supply to the heart muscle is reduced. *See Atherosclerosis.*

CORONARY OCCLUSION

An obstruction (generally a blood clot) in a branch of one of the coronary arteries which hinders the flow of blood to some part of the heart muscle. This part of the heart muscle then dies because of lack of blood supply. Sometimes called a coronary heart attack, or simply a heart attack.

CORONARY THROMBOSIS

Formation of a clot in a branch of one of the arteries which conduct blood to the heart muscle (coronary arteries). A form of coronary occlusion. *See Coronary Occlusion.*

COR PULMONALE

Heart disease resulting from disease of the lungs or the blood vessels in the lungs. This is due to resistance to the passage of blood through the lungs.

CORVISART, JEAN NICOLAS (1755–1821)

One of earliest of the modern cardiologists, and the first man to call himself a "heart specialist." Favorite physician to Napoleon.

COUMARIN

A class of chemical substances which delay clotting of the blood. An anti-coagulant.

CRUDE DEATH RATE

Also called crude mortality rate. The ratio of total deaths to total population during a given period of time, such as a year. It is calculated by dividing the total number of deaths during the year by the mid-year population (estimated population on July 1) of the same year.

CYANOSIS

Blueness of skin caused by insufficient oxygen in the blood. Oxygen is carried in the blood by hemoglobin, which is bright red when saturated with oxygen. When hemoglobin is not carrying oxygen, it is purple and is called reduced hemoglobin. The blueness of the skin occurs when the amount of reduced hemoglobin exceeds 5 grams per 100 cc. of blood.

CYTOLOGIC

Pertaining to cells, their anatomy, physiology, pathology, and chemistry.

DECOMPENSATION

Inability of the heart to maintain adequate circulation, usually resulting in a waterlogging of tissues. A person whose heart is failing to maintain normal circulation is said to be "decompensated."

DEFIBRILLATOR

Any agent or measure, such as an electric shock, which stops an incoordinate contraction of the heart muscle and restores a normal heart beat.

DEPRESSANT

Any drug which decreases functional activity.

DESCARTES, RENE (1596–1650)

Author of the first physiology textbook which accepted the theory of the circulation of the blood as described by William Harvey.

DEXIOCARDIA

Same as dextrocardia.

DEXTROCARDIA

Two different types of congenital phenomena are often described as dextrocardia. The first is a condition in which the heart is slightly rotated and lies almost entirely in the right (instead of the left) side of the chest. The second is a condition in which there is a complete transposition, the left chambers of the heart being on the right side, and the right chambers on the left side, so that the heart presents a mirror image of the normal heart.

DIASTOLE

In each heart beat, the period of the relaxation of the heart. Auricular diastole is the period of relaxation of

162

the atria, or upper heart chambers. Ventricular diastole is the period of relaxation of the ventricles, or lower heart chambers.

DIET

Daily allowance or intake of food and drink.

DIETETICS

The science and art dealing with the application of principles of nutrition to the feeding of individuals or groups under different economic or health conditions.

DIETITIAN

One skilled in the scientific use of diet in health and disease.

DIGITALIS

A drug prepared from leaves of foxglove plant which strengthens the contraction of the heart muscle, slows the rate of contraction of the heart, and by improving the efficiency of the heart, may promote the elimination of fluid from body tissues.

DILATION

A stretching or enlargement of the heart or blood vessels beyond the norm.

DIURESIS

Increased excretion of urine.

DIURETIC
A medicine which promotes the excretion of urine. Several types of drugs may be used, such as mercurials, chlorothiazide, xanthine, and benzothiadiazine derivatives.

DUCTUS ARTERIOSUS
A small duct in the heart of the fetus between the artery leaving the left side of the heart (aorta) and the artery leaving the right side of the heart (pulmonary artery). Normally this duct closes soon after birth. If it does not close, the condition is known as patent or open ductus arteriosus. *See Patent Ductus Arteriosus.*

DYSPNEA
Difficult or labored breathing.

ECG
See Electrocardiogram.

ECTOMORPH
Wiry body type.

EDEMA
Swelling due to abnormally large amounts of fluid in the tissues of the body.

EFFORT SYNDROME
A group of symptoms (quick fatigue, rapid heart beat, sighing breaths, dizziness) that do not result from

disease of organs or tissues and that are out of proportion to the amount of exertion required.

EKG

See Electrocardiogram.

ELECTRIC CARDIAC PACEMAKER

An electric device that can control the beating of the heart by a rhythmic discharge of electrical impulses.

ELECTROCARDIOGRAM

Often referred to as EKG or ECG. A graphic record of the electric currents produced by the heart.

ELECTROCARDIOGRAPH

An instrument which records electric currents produced by the heart.

ELECTROLYTE

Any substance which, in solution, is capable of conducting electricity by means of its atoms or groups of atoms, and in the process is broken down into positively and negatively charged particles. Examples, sodium or potassium.

EMBOLISM

The blocking of a blood vessel by a clot or other substance carried in the blood stream.

165

EMBOLUS

A blood clot (or other substance such as air, fat, tumor) inside a blood vessel which is carried in the blood stream to a smaller vessel where it becomes an obstruction to circulation. *See Thrombus.*

ENDARTERIUM

Also called intima. The innermost layer of an artery.

ENDOCARDITIS

Inflammation of the inner layer of the heart (endocardium) usually associated with acute rheumatic fever or some infectious agents.

ENDOCARDIUM

A thin smooth membrane forming the inner surface of the heart.

ENDOMORPH

Short and thickset body type.

ENDOTHELIUM

The thin lining of the blood vessels.

ENZYME

A complex organic substance which is capable of speeding up specific biochemical processes in the body. Enzymes are universally present in living organisms.

EPICARDIUM

The outer layer of the heart wall. Also called the visceral pericardium.

EPIDEMIOLOGY

The science dealing with the factors which determine the frequency and distribution of a disease in a human community.

EPINEPHRINE

One of the secretions of two small glands, called adrenal glands, located just above the kidneys. This secretion, also called adrenalin, and sometimes prepared synthetically, constricts the small blood vessels (arterioles), increases the rate of heart beat, and raises blood pressure. It is called a vasoconstrictor or vasopressor substance.

ERYTHROCYTE

Red blood cell.

ESSENTIAL HYPERTENSION

Sometimes called primary hypertension, and commonly known as high blood pressure. An elevated blood pressure not caused by kidney or other evident disease.

ETIOLOGY
The sum of knowledge about the causes of a disease.

EXTRACORPOREAL CIRCULATION
The circulation of the blood outside the body as by a mechanical pump-oxygenator. This is often done while surgery is being performed inside the heart.

EXTRASYSTOLE
A contraction of the heart which occurs prematurely and interrupts the normal rhythm.

EYEGROUND
The inside of the back part of the eye seen by looking through the pupil. Examining the eyeground is one means of assessing changes in the blood vessels. Also called the fundus of the eye.

FABRICIUS AB AQUAPENDENTE, HIERONYMUS (1560–1634)
Italian anatomist, a teacher of William Harvey at Padua. He studied the valves of the veins and Harvey is reported to have credited the work of Fabricius with leading to his own concept of the circulation of the blood.

FALLOT, ETIENNE LOUIS ARTHUR (1850–1911)
French physician who gave an important description of a congenital heart defect known as the tetralogy of Fallot. *See Tetralogy of Fallot.*

FEMORAL ARTERY

Main blood vessel supplying blood to the leg.

FIBRILLATION

Uncoordinated contractions of the heart muscle occurring when the individual muscle fibers take up
independent irregular contractions.

FIBRIN

An elastic protein which forms the essential portion
of a blood clot.

FIBRINOGEN

A soluble protein in the blood which, by the action of
certain enzymes, is converted into the insoluble protein of a blood clot.

FIBRINOLYSIN

An enzyme which can cause coagulated blood to return to a liquid state.

FIBRINOLYTIC

Having the ability to dissolve a blood clot.

FLUORESCENT ANTIBODY TEST

A rapid and sensitive test for certain disease organisms and substances. Its value in the field of heart
disease is that it speeds the recognition of harmful

streptococci in a throat smear, so that immediate treatment might avert an attack of rheumatic fever. The test consists of "tagging" with a fluorescent dye the antibodies, i.e., substances in blood serum that have been built up against certain bacteria. This dyed antibody is then mixed with a smear taken from the throat of the patient. If streptococci are present in the smear, the glowing antibodies will attach to them, and they can be clearly seen in the microscope.

FLUOROSCOPE
An instrument for observing structures deep inside the body. X-rays are passed through the body onto a fluorescent screen where the shadow of deep-lying organs can be seen.

FLUOROSCOPY
The examination of a structure deep in the body by means of observing the fluorescence of a screen caused by X-rays transmitted through the body.

FORAMEN OVALE
An oval hole between the left and right upper chambers of the heart which normally closes shortly after birth. Its failure to close is one of the congenital defects of the heart, called a patent foramen ovale.

FUNDUS OF THE EYE
The inside of the back part of the eye seen by looking through the pupil. Examining the fundus of the eye is

170

used as a means of assessing changes in the blood vessels. Also called the eyeground.

GALEN (CLAUDIUS GALENUS) (c. 130–200 A.D.)

Renowned Greek physician whose theory that life and health depended upon the balance of four "humors" in the body, dominated medical practice for 1500 years. His concept of the ebb and flow of the blood which transported the humors to various parts of the body, was not refuted until William Harvey's discovery of the circulation of the blood in 1628.

GALLOP RHYTHM

An extra, clearly heard heart sound which, when the heart rate is fast, resembles a horse's gallop. It may or may not be significant.

GANGLION

A mass of nerve cells, which serves as a center of nervous influence.

GANGLIONIC BLOCKING AGENTS

A drug that blocks the transmission of a nerve impulse at the nerve centers (ganglia). Some of these drugs, such as hexamethonium and mecamylamine hydrochloride, may be used in the treatment of high blood pressure.

GENETICS

The study of heredity.

HARVEY, WILLIAM (1578–1657)

English physician who discovered the circulation of the blood and described his theory in 1628 in his classic work *De Motu Cordis.*

HEART BLOCK

Interference with the conduction of the electrical impulses of the heart which can be either partial or complete. This can result in dissociation of the rhythms of the upper and lower heart chambers.

HEART-LUNG MACHINE

A machine through which the blood stream is diverted for pumping and oxygenation while the heart is opened for surgery. *See Extracorporeal Circulation.*

HEMIPLEGIA

Paralysis of one side of the body caused by damage to the opposite side of the brain. The paralyzed arm and leg are opposite to the side of the brain damage because the nerves cross in the brain, and one side of the brain controls the opposite side of the body. Such paralysis is sometimes caused by a blood clot or hemorrhage in a blood vessel in the brain. *See Stroke.*

HEMODYNAMICS

The study of the flow of blood and the forces involved.

HEMOGLOBIN

The oxygen-carrying red pigment of the red blood corpuscles. When it has absorbed oxygen in the lungs, it is bright red and called oxy-hemoglobin. After it has given up its oxygen load in the tissues, it is purple in color, and is called reduced hemoglobin.

HEMORRHAGE

Loss of blood from a blood vessel. In external hemorrhage blood escapes from the body. In internal hemorrhage blood passes into tissues surrounding the ruptured blood vessel.

HEPARIN

A chemical substance which tends to prevent blood from clotting. Sometimes used in cases of an existing clot in an artery or vein to prevent enlargement of the clot or the formation of new clots. An anticoagulant.

HEXAMETHONIUM CHLORIDE

A drug which lowers blood pressure and increases blood flow by interfering with the transmission of nerve impulses which constrict the blood vessels. One of the ganglionic blocking agents, it is one of the drugs used in the treatment of high blood pressure.

HIS, WILHELM (1831–1904)

German anatomist who discovered the bundle of muscle fibers running from the upper to lower chambers of heart. These fibers are known as "Bundle of His."

HISTOLOGY
> The study of the anatomy of the cells and minute structures of the tissues and organs.

HYDRALAZINE HYDROCHLORIDE
> A drug which lowers blood pressure. One of the antihypertensive agents.

HYPERCHOLESTEREMIA
> An excess of a fatty substance called cholesterol in the blood. Sometimes called hypercholesterolemia or hypercholesterinemia. *See Cholesterol.*

HYPERLIPEMIA
> An excess of fat or lipids in the blood.

HYPERTENSION
> Commonly called high blood pressure. An unstable or persistent elevation of blood pressure above the normal range, which may eventually lead to increased heart size and kidney damage. *See Primary Hypertension* and *Secondary Hypertension.*

HYPERTHYROIDISM
> A condition in which the thyroid gland is overly active. This may eventually result in a speeded up rate of heart beat.

HYPERTROPHY
>   The enlargement of a tissue or organ due to increase in the size of its constituent cells. This may result from a demand for increased work.

HYPOTENSION
>   Commonly called low blood pressure. Blood pressure below the normal range. Most commonly used to describe an acute fall in blood pressure, as occurs in shock.

HYPOTHALAMUS
>   A part of the brain which exerts control over activity of the abdominal organs, water balance, temperature, etc. Damage to the hypothalamus may cause abnormal gain in weight, among other things.

HYPOTHERMIA
>   Also called hypothermy. The lowering of the body temperature (usually to 86°—88°F.) in order to slow the metabolic processes during heart surgery. In this cooled state, body tissues require less oxygen.

HYPOTHYROIDISM
>   A condition in which the thyroid gland is underactive, resulting in the slowing down of many of the body processes including the heart rate.

HYPOXIA

Less than normal content of oxygen in the organs and tissues of the body. At very high altitudes a healthy person suffers from hypoxia because of insufficient oxygen in the air that is breathed.

IATROGENIC HEART DISEASE

Literally means "caused by the doctor." A patient's belief that he has heart disease implied from the actions, manner, or discussions of the physician or some member of the medical team.

ILIAC ARTERY

A large artery which conducts blood to the pelvis and the legs.

INCIDENCE

The number of new cases of a disease developing in a given population during a specified period of time, such as a year.

INCOMPETENT VALVE

Any valve which does not close tight and leaks blood back in the wrong direction. Also called valvular insufficiency.

INFARCT

An area of a tissue which is damaged or dies as a result of not receiving a sufficient blood supply. Frequently used in the phrase "myocardial infarct" referring to an area of the heart muscle damaged or killed by an insufficient flow of blood through the coronary arteries which normally supply it.

INNOMINATE ARTERY

One of the largest branches of the aorta. It arises from the arch of the aorta and divides to form the right common carotid artery and the right subclavian artery.

INSUFFICIENCY

Incompetency. In the term "valvular insufficiency," an improper closing of the valves which admits a back flow of blood in the wrong direction. In the term "myocardial insufficiency," inability of the heart muscle to do a normal pumping job.

INTER-ATRIAL SEPTUM

Sometimes called auricular septum or interauricular septum or atrial septum. Muscular wall dividing left and right upper chambers of the heart which are called atria.

INTER-VENTRICULAR SEPTUM

Sometimes called ventricular septum. Muscular wall, thinner at the top, dividing the left and right lower chambers of the heart which are called ventricles.

INTIMA

The innermost layer of a blood vessel.

IN VITRO

Literally means "in glass," hence in a laboratory vessel. Describes a phenomenon studied outside a living body under laboratory conditions. *See In Vivo.*

IN VIVO

In a living organism. Describes a phenomenon studied in a living body. *See In Vitro.*

ISCHEMIA

A local, usually temporary, deficiency of blood in some part of the body, often caused by a constriction or an obstruction in the blood vessel supplying that part.

ISOTOPE

A term applied to one of two elements, chemically identical, but differing in some other characteristic, such as radioactivity. Radioactive isotopes are often used in medicine to trace the fate of substances in the body.

JUGULAR VEINS

Veins which return blood from the head and neck to the heart.

LAENNEC, RENE THEOPHILE HYACINTHE (1781–1826)
French physician who invented the stethoscope.

LEEUWENHOEK, ANTONN J. VAN (1632–1723)
Dutch microscopist who, among other scientific contributions, discovered the interwoven structure of the muscle fibers of the heart.

LEVARTERENOL
One of the normal secretions of the adrenal glands, and also a drug. It raises blood pressure and is used to treat acute low blood pressure and shock.

LINOLEIC ACID
An important component of many of the unsaturated fats. It is found widely in oils from plants. A diet with a high linoleic acid content tends to lower the amount of cholesterol in the blood.

LIPID
Fat.

LIPOPROTEIN
A complex of fat and protein molecules.

LUMEN
The passageway inside a tubular organ. Vascular lumen is the passageway inside a blood vessel.

MALIGNANT HYPERTENSION
Severe high blood pressure that runs a rapid course and causes damage to the blood vessel walls in the kidney, eye, etc.

MALPIGHI, MARCELLO (1628–1694)
Italian anatomist who, among other discoveries, demonstrated the existence of capillary connections between the arteries and veins in the lungs.

MECAMYLAMINE HYDROCHLORIDE
A drug which blocks the transmission of nerve impulses at the nerve centers. One of the ganglionic blocking agents, it may be used in the treatment of high blood pressure.

MERCURIAL DIURETIC
Various organic compounds of mercury commonly used to promote the elimination of water and sodium from the body through increased excretion of urine. Sometimes used in congestive heart failure when tissues are water-logged. Mercury in several different organic forms is used as a diuretic.

MESOMORPH
Muscular body type.

METABOLISM
A general term to designate all chemical changes which occur to substances within the body.

MITRAL INSUFFICIENCY

An improper closing of the mitral valve between the upper and lower chambers in the left side of the heart which admits a back flow of blood in the wrong direction. Sometimes the result of scar tissue forming after a rheumatic fever infection.

MITRAL STENOSIS

A narrowing of the valve (called bicuspid or mitral valve) opening between the upper and the lower chambers in the left side of the heart. Sometimes the result of scar tissue forming after a rheumatic fever infection.

MITRAL VALVE

Sometimes called bicuspid valve. A valve of two cusps or triangular segments, located between the upper and lower chambers in the left side of the heart.

MITRAL VALVULOTOMY

An operation to widen the opening in the valve between the upper and lower chambers in the left side of the heart (mitral valve). Usually performed when the valve opening is so narrowed as to obstruct blood flow, which sometimes happens as a result of rheumatic fever.

MONO-UNSATURATED FAT

A fat so constituted chemically that it is capable of absorbing additional hydrogen but not as much hydrogen as a poly-unsaturated fat. These fats in the diet have little effect on the amount of cholesterol in the blood. One example is olive oil. *See Polyunsaturated Fat.*

MORBIDITY RATE

The ratio of the number of cases of a disease to the number of well people in a given population during a specified period of time, such as a year. The term "morbidity" involves two separate concepts.

a. Incidence is the number of new cases of a disease developing in a given population during a specified period of time, such as a year.

b. Prevalence is the number of cases of a given disease existing in a given population at a specified moment of time.

MORTALITY RATE—AGE-ADJUSTED

Also called age-adjusted death rate. Death rates which have been standardized for age for the purpose of making comparisons between different populations or within the same population at various intervals of time. The age-specific death rates of the populations being compared are applied to a population that is arbitrarily selected as standard, to determine what would be the crude death rate in the standard population if it were exposed first to the rates of the one population and then to the rates of the other.

MORTALITY RATE—AGE-SPECIFIC

Also called age-specific death rate. The ratio of deaths in a specific age group to the population of the same age group during a given period of time, such as a year. It is calculated by dividing the deaths that occurred among the specific age group during the year by the mid-year population in the same group (estimated population in the age group on July 1) of the same year.

MORTALITY RATE—CAUSE-SPECIFIC
The ratio of deaths from a specific cause to total population during a given period of time, such as a year.

MORTALITY RATE—CRUDE
The ratio of total deaths to total population during a given period of time, such as a year. Sometimes called crude death rate. It is calculated by dividing the total number of deaths during the year by the mid-year population (estimated population of July 1) of the same year.

MORTALITY RATE (SPECIFIC-CAUSE-OF-DEATH)
The number of deaths from a specific cause that occurred in a unit of population (such as per 100,000 or per 10,000 or per 1,000) in a specified time, such as a year.

MURMUR
An abnormal heart sound, sounding like fluid passing an obstruction, heard between the normal lub-dub heart sounds.

183

MYOCARDIAL INFARCTION
The damaging or death of an area of the heart muscle (myocardium) resulting from a reduction in the blood supply reaching that area.

MYOCARDIAL INSUFFICIENCY
An inability of the heart muscle (myocardium) to maintain normal circulation. *See Congestive Heart Failure.*

MYOCARDITIS
Inflammation of the heart muscle (myocardium).

MYOCARDIUM
The muscular wall of the heart. The thickest of the three layers of the heart wall, it lies between the inner layer (endocardium) and the outer layer (epicardium).

NEUROCIRCULATORY ASTHENIA
Sometimes called soldier's heart or effort syndrome. A complex of nervous and circulatory symptoms, often involving a sense of fatigue, dizziness, shortness of breath, rapid heart beat, and nervousness. *See Effort Syndrome.*

NEUROGENIC
Originating in the nervous system.

NEUROSIS
>A functional nervous disease in which the personality remains more or less intact.

NITRITES
>A group of chemical compounds, many of which cause dilation of the small blood vessels, and thus lower blood pressure. They are vasodilators. Examples are amyl nitrite, sodium nitrite, etc.

NITROGLYCERIN
>A drug (one of the nitrates) which relaxes the muscles in the blood vessels. Often used to relieve attacks of angina pectoris and spasm of coronary arteries. It is one of the vasodilators.

NORADRENALIN
>An organic compound which produces a rise in blood pressure by constricting the small blood vessels. Sometimes used in the treatment of shock. Also called norepinephrine and levarterenol.

NOREPINEPHRINE
>An organic compound which produces a rise in blood pressure by constricting the small blood vessels. Sometimes used in the treatment of shock. Also called noradrenalin and levarterenol.

NORMOTENSIVE
>Characterized by normal blood pressure.

NUTRITION
> The combination of processes by which a living organism receives and utilizes the materials necessary for the maintenance of its functions and for the growth and renewal of its components.

NUTRITIONIST
> One professionally engaged in investigating and solving problems of nutrition.

OPEN HEART SURGERY
> Surgery performed on the opened heart while the blood stream is diverted through a heart-lung machine. This machine pumps and oxygenates the blood in lieu of the action of the heart and lungs during the operation.

ORGANIC HEART DISEASE
> Heart disease caused by some structural abnormality in the heart or circulatory system.

OSCILLOMETER
> An instrument which measures the changes in magnitude of the pulsations in the arteries. Especially useful in studying circulation in the periphery of the body.

OTITIS MEDIA
> An infection of the middle ear, frequently caused by a spreading of a bacterial infection from the throat.

PACEMAKER

A small mass of specialized cells in the right upper chamber of the heart which give rise to the electrical impulses that initiate contractions of the heart. Also called sino-atrial node or S-A node of Keith-Flack. The term "pacemaker," or more exactly, "electric cardiac pacemaker," or "electrical pacemaker" is applied to an electrical device which can substitute for a defective natural pacemaker and control the beating of the heart by a series of rhythmic electrical discharges. If the electrodes which deliver the discharges to the heart are placed on the outside of the chest, it is called an "external pacemaker." If the electrodes are placed within the chest wall, it is called an "internal pacemaker."

PALPITATION

A fluttering of the heart or abnormal rate or rhythm of the heart experienced by the person himself.

PANCARDITIS

Inflammation of the whole heart including inner layer (endocardium), heart muscle (myocardium), and outer sac (pericardium).

PAPILLARY MUSCLES

Small bundles of muscles in the wall of the lower chambers of the heart to which the cords leading to the cusps of the valves (chordae tendineae) are attached. When the valves are closed, these muscles contract and tighten the cords which hold the valve firmly shut.

PARAPLEGIA

Loss of both motion and sensation in the legs and lower part of the body. This most commonly is due to damage to the spinal cord, but sometimes results from a blood clot or hemorrhage in an artery conducting blood to the spinal cord.

PARASYMPATHETIC NERVOUS SYSTEM

A part of the autonomic or involuntary nervous system. Stimulation of various parasympathetic nerves causes the pupils of the eyes to contract, the heart to beat more slowly, and produces other non-voluntary reactions.

PARIETAL PERICARDIUM

A thin membrane sac which surrounds the heart and roots of the great vessels. It is the outer layer of the pericardium.

PAROXYSMAL TACHYCARDIA

A period of rapid heart beats which begins and ends suddenly.

PATENT DUCTUS ARTERIOSUS

A congenital heart defect in which a small duct between the artery leaving the left side of the heart (aorta) and the artery leaving the right side of the heart (pulmonary artery), which normally closes soon after birth, remains open. As a result of this duct's failure to close, blood from both sides of the heart is pumped into the pulmonary artery and into the lungs. This defect is sometimes called simply patent ductus. Patent means open.

PATENT FORAMEN OVALE

One type of congenital heart defect. An oval hole between the left and right upper chambers of the heart, which normally closes shortly after birth, remains open.

PATHOGENESIS

The chain of events leading to the development of disease.

PATHOLOGY

The study of the essential nature of disease and the structural and functional changes it causes.

PERCUSSION

Tapping the body as an aid in diagnosing the condition of parts beneath by the sound obtained, much as one taps on a barrel to detect its fullness.

PERICARDITIS

Inflammation of the thin membrane sac (pericardium) which surrounds the heart.

PERICARDIUM

A thin membrane sac which surrounds the heart and roots of the great vessels.

189

PERIPHERAL RESISTANCE

The resistance offered by the arterioles and capillaries to the flow of blood from the arteries to the veins. An increase in peripheral resistance causes a rise in blood pressure.

PHARMACOLOGY

The science which deals with the study of drugs in all its aspects.

PHLEBITIS

Inflammation of a vein, often in the leg. Sometimes a blood clot is formed in the inflamed vein.

PHYSICAL THERAPY

The treatment of disease by physical means. Includes the use of heat, cold, water, light, electricity, manipulation, massage, exercise, and mechanical devices. Also called physiotherapy.

PLASMA

The cell-free liquid portion of uncoagulated blood. It is different from serum which is the fluid portion of the blood obtained after coagulation.

POLYCYTHEMIA

An abnormal condition of the blood characterized by an excessive number of red blood cells.

POLYGRAPH
> An instrument for taking synchronous records of several different pulsations.

POLY-UNSATURATED FAT
> A fat so constituted chemically that it is capable of absorbing additional hydrogen. These fats are usually liquid oils of vegetable origin, such as corn oil or safflower oil. A diet with a high poly-unsaturated fat content tends to lower the amount of cholesterol in the blood. These fats are sometimes substituted for saturated fat in a diet in an effort to lessen the hazard of fatty deposits in the blood vessels. *See Monounsaturated Fat.*

PRESSOR
> A substance which raises the blood pressure and accelerates the heart beat. Also denotes certain nerve fibers which produce a rise in blood pressure when stimulated.

PREVALENCE
> The number of cases of a given disease existing in a given population at a specified moment of time.

PRIMARY HYPERTENSION
> Sometimes called essential hypertension, and commonly known as high blood pressure. An elevated blood pressure not caused by kidney or other evident disease.

PROCAINE AMIDE
A drug sometimes used to treat abnormal rhythms of the heart beat.

PROPHYLAXIS
Preventive treatment.

PSYCHOSIS
A severe, specific mental disorder that has a characteristic origin, course, and symptoms.

PSYCHOSOMATIC
Pertaining to the influence of the mind, emotions, fears, etc. upon the functions of the body, especially in relation to disease.

PSYCHOTHERAPY
The treatment of disorders by the use of such means as persuasion, suggestion, educational techniques, lay or religious counseling, or psychoanalysis.

PULMONARY ARTERY
The large artery which conveys unoxygenated (venous) blood from the lower right chamber of the heart to the lungs. This is the only artery in the body which carries unoxygenated blood, all others carrying oxygenated blood to the body.

PULMONARY CIRCULATION

The circulation of the blood through the lungs, the flow being from the right lower chamber of the heart (right ventricle) through the lungs, back to the left upper chamber of the heart (left atrium). *See Systemic Circulation.*

PULMONARY VALVE

Valve, formed by three cup-shaped membranes at the junction of the pulmonary artery and the right lower chamber of the heart (right ventricle). When the right lower chamber contracts, the pulmonary valve opens and the blood is forced into the artery leading to the lungs. When the chamber relaxes, the valve is closed and prevents a back-flow of the blood.

PULMONARY VEINS

Four veins (two from each lung) which conduct oxygenated blood from the lungs into the left upper chamber of the heart (left atrium).

PULSE

The expansion and contraction of an artery which may be felt with the finger.

PULSE PRESSURE

The difference between the blood pressure in the arteries when the heart is in contraction (systole) and when it is in relaxation (diastole).

193

PULSUS ALTERNANS

A pulse in which there is regular alternation of weak and strong beats.

PURKINJE FIBERS

Specialized muscular fibers forming a network in the walls of the lower chambers of the heart and believed to be involved in conducting electrical impulses to the muscular walls of the two lower chambers (ventricles). These electrical impulses are responsible for the contractions of the heart.

QUINIDINE

A drug sometimes used to treat abnormal rhythms of the heart beat.

RAUWOLFIA

A drug consisting of powdered whole root of a plant (Rauwolfia serpentina) which lowers blood pressure and slows the heart rate. Sometimes used in treatment of high blood pressure. An antihypertensive agent. *See Reserpine.*

REGURGITATION

The backward flow of blood through a defective valve.

REHABILITATION

The return of a person disabled by accident or disease to the maximum attainable physical, mental, emotional, social and economic usefulness, and, if employable, an opportunity for gainful employment.

RENAL

Pertaining to the kidney.

RENAL CIRCULATION

The circulation of the blood through the kidneys. Important in heart disease because of its function in the elimination of water, certain chemical elements, and waste products from the body.

RENAL HYPERTENSION

High blood pressure caused by damage to or disease of the kidneys.

RESERPINE

One of the organic substances found in the root of the plant, Rauwolfia serpentina, which lowers blood pressure, slows the heart rate, and has a sedative effect. One of the antihypertensive agents. *See Rauwolfia.*

RHEUMATIC FEVER

A disease, usually occurring in childhood, which may follow a few weeks after a streptococcal infection. It is sometimes characterized by one or more of the following: fever, sore swollen joints, a skin rash, occasionally by involuntary twitching of the muscles (called chorea or St. Vitus Dance) and small nodes under the skin. In some cases the infection affects the heart and may result in scarring the valves, weakening the heart muscle, or damaging the sac enclosing the heart. *See Rheumatic Heart Disease.*

RHEUMATIC HEART DISEASE
The damage done to the heart, particularly the heart valves, by one or more attacks of rheumatic fever. The valves are sometimes scarred so they do not open and close normally. *See Rheumatic Fever.*

RIOLAN, JEAN (1577–1657)
Dean of Faculty of Medicine at Paris, a staunch adherent to the old classical (Galen) theory of anatomy, he was one of the most active opponents of William Harvey who discovered the circulation of the blood.

S-A NODE
A small mass of specialized cells in the right upper chamber of the heart which gives rise to the electrical impulses that initiate contractions of the heart. Also called sino-atrial node or pacemaker.

SATURATED FAT
A fat so constituted chemically that it is not capable of absorbing any more hydrogen. These are usually the solid fats of animal origin such as the fats in milk, butter, meat, etc. A diet high in saturated fat content tends to increase the amount of cholesterol in the

blood. Sometimes these fats are restricted in the diet in an effort to lessen the hazard of fatty deposits in the blood vessels.

SCLEROSIS

Hardening, usually due to an accumulation of fibrous tissue.

SECONDARY HYPERTENSION

An elevated blood pressure caused by (i.e., secondary to) certain specific diseases or infections.

SEDATIVE

A drug which depresses the activity of the central nervous system, thus having a calming effect. Examples are barbiturates, chloral hydrate, and bromides.

SEMILUNAR VALVES

Cup-shaped valves. The aortic valve at the entrance to the aorta, and the pulmonary valve at the entrance to the pulmonary artery are semilunar valves. They consist of three cup-shaped flaps which prevent the back flow of blood.

SEPTUM

A dividing wall.

1. Atrial or inter-atrial septum. Muscular wall dividing left and right upper chambers (called atria) of the heart.

197

2. Ventricular or inter-ventricular septum. Muscular wall, thinner at the top, dividing the left and right lower chambers (called ventricles) of the heart.

SEROTONIN

A naturally occurring compound found mainly in the gastrointestinal tract and in lesser amounts in the blood, which has a stimulating effect on the circulatory system.

SERUM

The fluid portion of blood which remains after the cellular elements have been removed by coagulation. It is different from plasma which is the cell-free liquid portion of uncoagulated blood.

SERVETUS, MICHAEL (1509–1553)

Spanish physician who discovered the circulation of the blood through the lungs. Burned at the stake in Geneva for his religious doctrines.

SHUNT

A passage between two blood vessels or between the two sides of the heart, as in cases where an opening exists in the wall which normally separates them. In surgery, the operation of forming a passage between blood vessels to divert blood from one part of the body to another.

SIGN

Any objective evidence of a disease. *See Symptom.*

SINO-ATRIAL NODE

A small mass of specialized cells in the right upper chamber of the heart which give rise to the electrical impulses that initiate contractions of the heart. Also called S-A node or pacemaker.

SINUSES OF VALSALVA

Three pouches in the wall of the aorta (main artery leading from left lower chamber of the heart) behind the three cup-shaped membranes of the aortic valve.

SODIUM

A mineral essential to life, found in nearly all plant and animal tissue. Table salt (sodium chloride) is nearly half sodium. In some types of heart disease the body retains an excess of sodium and water, and therefore sodium intake is restricted.

SPHYGMOMANOMETER

An instrument for measuring blood pressure in the arteries.

STASIS

A stoppage or slackening of the blood flow.

STENOSIS

A narrowing or stricture of an opening. Mitral stenosis, aortic stenosis, etc. means that the valve indicated has become narrowed so that it does not function normally.

STETHOSCOPE

An instrument for listening to sounds within the body.

STOKES-ADAMS SYNDROME

Sudden attacks of unconsciousness, sometimes with convulsions, which may accompany heart block.

STROKE

Also called apoplectic stroke, cerebrovascular accident, or cerebral vascular accident. An impeded blood supply to some part of the brain, generally caused by:

1. a blood clot forming in the vessel (cerebral thrombosis)

2. a rupture of the blood vessel wall (cerebral hemorrhage)

3. a piece of clot or other material from another part of the vascular system which flows to the brain and obstructs a cerebral vessel (cerebral embolism)

4. pressure on a blood vessel, as by a tumor.

STROKE VOLUME

The amount of blood which is pumped out of the heart at each contraction of the heart.

SYMPATHECTOMY

An operation which interrupts some part of the sympathetic nervous system. The sympathetic nervous system is a part of the autonomic or involuntary nervous system and normally regulates tissues not under voluntary control, e.g., glands, heart, and smooth muscles. Sometimes the interruption is accomplished by drugs, in which case it is called a chemical sympathectomy.

SYMPATHETIC NERVOUS SYSTEM

A part of the autonomic nervous system or involuntary nervous system, it regulates tissues not under voluntary control, e.g., glands, heart, and smooth muscle. *See Parasympathetic Nervous System.*

SYMPTOM

Any subjective evidence of a patient's condition. *See Sign.*

SYNCOPE

A faint. One cause for syncope can be an insufficient blood supply to the brain.

SYNDROME

A set of symptoms which occur together and are therefore given a name to indicate that particular combination.

SYSTEMIC CIRCULATION

The circulation of the blood through all parts of the body except the lungs, the flow being from the left lower chamber of the heart (left ventricle) through the body, back to the right upper chamber of the heart (right atrium). *See Pulmonary Circulation.*

SYSTOLE

In each heart beat, the period of contraction of the heart. Atrial systole is the period of the contraction of the upper chambers of the heart, called the atria.

Ventricular systole is the period of the contraction of the lower chambers of the heart, called the ventricles.

TACHYCARDIA

Abnormally fast heart rate. Generally, anything over 100 beats per minute is considered a tachycardia.

TETRALOGY OF FALLOT

A congenital malformation of the heart involving four distinct defects (hence tetralogy). Named for Etienne Fallot, French physician who described the condition in 1888. The four defects are:

1. an abnormal opening in the wall between the lower chambers of the heart

2. misplacement of the aorta, "over-riding" the abnormal opening, so that it receives blood from both the right and left lower chambers instead of only the left
3. narrowing of the pulmonary artery
4. enlargement of the right lower chamber of the heart.

THERAPIST
A person skilled in the treatment of disease.

THIOCYANATE
A chemical which causes dilation of the small blood vessels, thus lowering blood pressure. It is a vasodilator.

THROMBECTOMY
An operation to remove a blood clot from a blood vessel.

THROMBOLYTIC AGENTS
Substance which dissolve blood clots.

THROMBOPHLEBITIS
Inflammation and blood clotting in a vein.

THROMBOSIS

The formation or presence of a blood clot (thrombus) inside a blood vessel or cavity of the heart.

THROMBUS

A blood clot which forms inside a blood vessel or cavity of the heart. *See Embolus.*

THYROTOXIC

Pertaining to overactivity or abnormal activity of the thyroid gland.

TOXEMIA

The condition caused by poisonous substances in the blood.

TOXIC

Pertaining to poison.

TRICUSPID VALVE

A valve consisting of three cusps or triangular segments located between the upper and lower chamber in the right side of the heart. Its position corresponds to the bicuspid or mitral valve in the left side of the heart.

UREMIA

An excess in the blood of certain waste substances normally excreted by the kidneys.

VAGUS NERVES

Two of the nerves of the parasympathetic nervous system which extend from the brain, through the neck and thorax into the abdomen. Known as the inhibitory nerves of the heart, they slow the heart rate when stimulated.

VALVULAR INSUFFICIENCY

Valves which close improperly and admit a back flow of blood in the wrong direction. *See Incompetent Valve.*

VASOCONSTRICTOR

The vasoconstrictor nerves are one part of the involuntary nervous system. When these nerves are stimulated they cause the muscles of the arterioles to contract, thus narrowing the arteriole passage, increasing the resistance to the flow of blood, and raising the blood pressure. Chemical substances which stimulate the muscles of the arterioles to contract are called vasoconstrictor agents or vasopressors. An example is adrenalin or epinephrine.

VASODILATOR

Vasodilator nerves are certain nerve fibers of the involuntary nervous system which cause the muscles of the arterioles to relax, thus enlarging the arteriole passage, reducing resistance to the flow of blood, and lowering blood pressure.

Vasodilator agents are chemical compounds which

cause a relaxation of the muscles of the arterioles. Examples of this type of drug are nitroglycerine, nitrites, thiocyanate, and many others.

VASO-INHIBITOR

An agent or drug which inhibits the action of the vasomotor nerves. When these involuntary nerves are inhibited, the muscles of the arterioles relax, and the passage inside the arteriole is enlarged, and the blood pressure is lowered. Examples of this type of drug are compounds of nitrite.

VASOPRESSOR

A chemical substance which causes the muscles of the arterioles to contract, narrowing the arteriole passage, and thus raises the blood pressure. Such substances are also called vasoconstrictors. An example is adrenalin or epinephrine.

VECTORCARDIOGRAPHY

Determination of the direction and magnitude of the electrical forces of the heart.

VEIN

Any one of a series of vessels of the vascular system which carries blood from various parts of the body back to the heart. All veins in the body conduct unoxygenated blood except the pulmonary veins which conduct freshly oxygenated blood from the lungs back to the heart.

VENA CAVA

Superior vena cava is a large vein conducting blood from the upper part of the body (head, neck, and thorax) to the right upper chamber of the heart. Inferior vena cava is a large vein conducting blood from the lower part of the body to the right upper chamber of the heart.

VENOUS BLOOD

Unoxygenated blood. The blood, with hemoglobin in the reduced state, is carried by the veins from all parts of the body back to the heart and then pumped by the right side of the heart to the lungs where it is oxygenated.

VENTRICLE

One of the two lower chambers of the heart. Left ventricle pumps oxygenated blood through arteries to the body. Right ventricle pumps unoxygenated blood through pulmonary artery to lungs. Capacity about 85 cc.

VENTRICULAR SEPTUM

Sometimes called inter-ventricular septum. Muscular wall, thinner at the top, dividing the left and right lower chambers of the heart which are called ventricles. *See Septum.*

VENULE

A very small vein.

VERATRUM

A drug which lowers blood pressure and decreases the heart rate. One of the anti-hypertensive agents.

VESALIUS, ANDREAS (1514–1564)

Belgian anatomist who questioned many of the then current theories of the circulatory system as taught by Galen, chiefly the existence of openings in the wall dividing the left from the right side of the heart through which blood was believed to pass.

VISCERAL PERICARDIUM

The outer layer of the heart wall. Also called the "epicardium."

WITHERING, WILLIAM (1741–1799)

Eminent English clinician who discovered the use and proper dosage of digitalis in the treatment of heart disease. By analyzing the effective herbal mixture used by an old woman in Shropshire, he identified foxglove leaves as the active ingredient which influenced the function of the heart and kidneys.

WORK CLASSIFICATION UNIT

A community facility involving a team approach to assessing the ability of the cardiac patient to work in terms of the energy requirements of the job.

XANTHINE

A class of drugs used to increase the excretion of urine. A diuretic.